Zebrafish Models for Experimental Pharmacology: A Handbook

Edited by

Shamsher Singh
Neuropharmacology Division
Department of Pharmacology
ISF College of Pharmacy
Moga, Punjab 142001, India

Zebrafish Models for Experimental Pharmacology: A Handbook

Editor: Shamsher Singh

ISBN (Online): 978-981-5324-63-1

ISBN (Print): 978-981-5324-64-8

ISBN (Paperback): 978-981-5324-65-5

need for a court order if at any point you breach any terms of this License Agreement. In no event will any delay or failure by Bentham Science Publishers in enforcing your compliance with this License Agreement constitute a waiver of any of its rights.

3. You acknowledge that you have read this License Agreement, and agree to be bound by its terms and conditions. To the extent that any other terms and conditions presented on any website of Bentham Science Publishers conflict with, or are inconsistent with, the terms and conditions set out in this License Agreement, you acknowledge that the terms and conditions set out in this License Agreement shall prevail.

Bentham Science Publishers Pte. Ltd.
No. 9 Raffles Place
Office No. 26-01
Singapore 048619
Singapore
Email: subscriptions@benthamscience.net

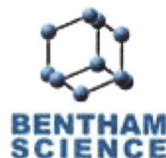

BENTHAM SCIENCE

CONTENTS

FOREWORD i

PREFACE ii

INTRODUCTION iii

LIST OF CONTRIBUTORS v

CHAPTER 1 INTRODUCTION AND BASICS TO ZEBRAFISH 1
Omkar Kumar Kuwar, Kousik Maparu and *Shamsher Singh*
INTRODUCTION 1
ZEBRAFISH MAINTENANCE 2
FEEDING 4
BREEDING 5
   Caring of Larvae 6
ZEBRAFISH AS A MODEL 7
   Toxicity Analysis 9
      Ocular Toxicity 9
      Neurotoxicity 11
      Embryotoxicity 11
      Cardiovascular Toxicity 12
      Toxicity in other organs 12
   Benefits of using Zebrafish as a Model 12
   Limitations of using Zebrafish as a Model 13
   Application of Zebrafish as an Experimental Model 13
PRACTICE QUESTIONS 13
REFERENCES 14

CHAPTER 2 ROUTES OF DRUG ADMINISTRATION IN ZEBRAFISH 16
Kousik Maparu and *Shamsher Singh*
INTRODUCTION 16
REQUIREMENTS 17
PROCEDURES 17
   Intra-muscular (i.m.) 17
   Intra-peritoneal (i.p.) 18
   Intrathoracic 20
RESULT 21
APPLICATIONS 21
ADVANTAGES 21
LIMITATIONS 21
FUTURE DIRECTIONS 22
PRACTICE QUESTIONS 22
REFERENCES 22

CHAPTER 3 BLOOD COLLECTION METHODS IN ZEBRAFISH 23
Nileshwar Kalia, Ayansh Kaushik and *Shamsher Singh*
INTRODUCTION 23
REQUIREMENTS 24
PROCEDURE 24
   Tail Transection Method 24
      Method of Anesthesia 24
   Cardiac Puncture Method 26

Micro-Capillary Tube Method from Dorsal Aorta 26
APPLICATIONS 27
LIMITATIONS 28
PRACTICE QUESTIONS 28
REFERENCES 28

CHAPTER 4 ANESTHESIA TECHNIQUES IN ZEBRAFISH 30
Kousik Maparu, Falguni Goel and *Shamsher Singh*
INTRODUCTION 30
    Stages of Anesthesia in Zebrafish 31
    Commonly Used Anesthetic Agents 32
REQUIREMENTS 33
GENERAL PROCEDURE FOR ANESTHESIA 33
ANESTHETIC TECHNIQUES 33
    Immersion Anesthesia 33
    Inhalation Anesthesia 34
    Anesthesia by Cooling 34
MONITORING AND SAFETY 35
CONSIDERATIONS 35
PRACTICE QUESTIONS 35
REFERENCES 36

CHAPTER 5 SHOALING BEHAVIOUR IN ZEBRAFISH 37
Pratyush Porel and *Shamsher Singh*
INTRODUCTION 37
REQUIREMENTS 38
SHOALING BEHAVIOUR IN ZEBRAFISH 38
    Factors Affecting the Shoaling Behavior in Zebrafish 40
        Temperature of Water 40
        pH of Water 41
        Tank Size 41
        Flow of Water 41
        Influence of Sex and Phenotype 42
    Research Outcomes on Shoaling Behaviour 42
        Alcohol 42
        Caffeine 42
        Quercetin 43
APPLICATIONS OF SHOALING BEHAVIOUR AND DISEASE CONDITIONS 43
ADVANTAGES 44
LIMITATIONS 44
PRACTICE QUESTIONS 45
REFERENCES 45

CHAPTER 6 ANIMAL MODELS OF ZEBRAFISH 47
Romanpreet Kaur and *Shamsher Singh*
INTRODUCTION 47
WHY ZEBRAFISH IS PREFERRED AS AN ANIMAL MODEL? 47
APPLICATIONS 48
SCOPE OF ZEBRAFISH 48
    Classification of Diseases in which Zebrafish are used as an Animal Model 49
        Metabolic Disorders 50
        Developmental Disorders 51

    Neurodegenerative Disorders 52

    Cancer 54

    Infections 55

    Cardiovascular Diseases 57

    Other Diseases 58

DRUG ADMINISTRATION IN ZEBRAFISH 58

    Methods of Drug Administration 58

ADVANTAGES 59

LIMITATIONS 59

FUTURE DIRECTIONS 59

CONCLUSION 59

PRACTICE QUESTIONS 60

REFERENCES 60

CHAPTER 7 NOVEL TANK DIVING TEST IN ZEBRAFISH 62

Falguni Goel, Romanpreet Kaur, Vaishali and *Shamsher Singh*

INTRODUCTION 62

REQUIREMENTS 63

PROCEDURE 63

    Parameters Measured 63

OBSERVATION 63

RESULT 64

APPLICATIONS 64

ADVANTAGES 65

LIMITATIONS 66

PRACTICE QUESTIONS 67

REFERENCES 67

CHAPTER 8 SOCIAL PREFERENCE TEST IN ZEBRAFISH 68

Falguni Goel, Mayank Attri, Khadga Raj and *Shamsher Singh*

INTRODUCTION 68

EXPERIMENTAL SETUP 69

REQUIREMENTS 70

PROCEDURE 70

    Data Analysis 71

OBSERVATION 71

RESULT 72

APPLICATIONS 72

ADVANTAGES 73

LIMITATIONS 73

PRACTICE QUESTIONS 74

REFERENCES 75

CHAPTER 9 MIRROR CHAMBER TEST IN ZEBRAFISH 76

Falguni Goel, Omkar Kumar Kuwar, Sania Grover and *Shamsher Singh*

INTRODUCTION 76

REQUIREMENTS 77

PROCEDURE 77

RESULT 79

APPLICATIONS 79

ADVANTAGES 80

LIMITATIONS 80

PRACTICE QUESTIONS 81
REFERENCES 81

CHAPTER 10 THREE-CHAMBER TEST IN ZEBRAFISH 83
Dhrita Chatterjee and *Shamsher Singh*
INTRODUCTION 83
REQUIREMENTS 83
PROCEDURE 84
OBSERVATION 84
RESULT 85
APPLICATIONS 86
ADVANTAGES 86
LIMITATIONS 86
PRACTICE QUESTIONS 86
REFERENCES 86

CHAPTER 11 LIGHT-DARK CHAMBER TEST IN ZEBRAFISH 87
Falguni Goel, Nileshwar Kalia, Lav Goyal and *Shamsher Singh*
INTRODUCTION 87
EXPERIMENTAL SETUP 88
REQUIREMENTS 89
PROCEDURE 89
OBSERVATION 90
RESULT 90
APPLICATIONS 91
ADVANTAGES 91
LIMITATIONS 92
PRACTICE QUESTIONS 92
REFERENCES 92

CHAPTER 12 PLUS-MAZE TEST IN ZEBRAFISH 94
Vaishali, Kousik Maparu and *Shamsher Singh*
INTRODUCTION 94
CONDITIONS OF THE ENVIRONMENT 94
    Evaluation Criteria 95
REQUIREMENTS 96
PROCEDURE 96
OBSERVATION 97
RESULT 98
APPLICATIONS 98
ADVANTAGES 98
LIMITATIONS 99
PRACTICE QUESTIONS 100
REFERENCES 100

CHAPTER 13 Y-MAZE TEST IN ZEBRAFISH 101
Dhrita Chatterjee, Kousik Maparu and *Shamsher Singh*
INTRODUCTION 101
REQUIREMENTS 102
PROCEDURE 102
    Data Analysis 103
CONDITIONS OF THE ENVIRONMENT 103
OBSERVATION 104

RESULT 105
APPLICATIONS 105
ADVANTAGES 105
LIMITATIONS 106
PRACTICE QUESTIONS 106
REFERENCES 106

CHAPTER 14 SQUARE-MAZE TEST IN ZEBRAFISH 107
Falguni Goel, Lovekesh Singh and *Shamsher Singh*
INTRODUCTION 107
EXPERIMENTAL CONSIDERATIONS 107
CONDITIONS OF THE ENVIRONMENT 107
    Parameters Measured 108
REQUIREMENTS 108
PROCEDURE 109
OBSERVATION 110
RESULT 110
APPLICATIONS 111
    Behavioral Insights 111
    Visual and Spatial Cues 111
ADVANTAGES 111
    Versatility 111
    Quantifiable Measures 111
    Standardization 111
    Ease of Use 112
    Non-invasive Observation 112
    Applicability to High-Throughput Screening 112
LIMITATIONS 112
    Limited Naturalistic Environment 112
    Spatial Constraints 112
    Data Interpretation 112
    Experimental Control 113
    Limited Task Variety 113
    Comparison with other Models 113
PRACTICE QUESTIONS 113
REFERENCES 114

CHAPTER 15 NOVEL OBJECT RECOGNITION TASK IN ZEBRAFISH 115
Dhrita Chatterjee and *Shamsher Singh*
INTRODUCTION 115
REQUIREMENTS 116
PROCEDURE 116
    Conditions of the Environment 117
OBSERVATION 117
RESULT 118
APPLICATIONS 118
ADVANTAGES 119
LIMITATIONS 119
PRACTICE QUESTIONS 119
REFERENCES 120

CHAPTER 16 OPEN FIELD TEST IN ZEBRAFISH 121

Mayank Attri, Anupam Awasthi and *Shamsher Singh*
INTRODUCTION 121
REQUIREMENTS 122
PROCEDURE 123
OBSERVATION 123
RESULT 124
APPLICATIONS 124
ADVANTAGES 125
LIMITATIONS 126
PRACTICE QUESTIONS 126
REFERENCES 126

CHAPTER 17 T-MAZE TEST IN ZEBRAFISH 127
Kousik Maparu, Vaishali, Dilpreet Kaur and *Shamsher Singh*
INTRODUCTION 127
REQUIREMENTS 128
PROCEDURE 128
Conditions of the Environment 129
OBSERVATION 129
RESULT 130
APPLICATIONS 130
ADVANTAGES 131
LIMITATIONS 131
PRACTICE QUESTIONS 131
REFERENCES 132

CHAPTER 18 LEARNING TEST IN ZEBRAFISH 133
Romanpreet Kaur and *Shamsher Singh*
INTRODUCTION 133
TYPES OF LEARNING 133
Non-associative learning 133
Associative Learning 134
Classical (Pavlovian) Conditioning 134
Operant (Instrumental) Conditioning 134
Other Types of Learning 134
Behavioral Learning in Zebrafish 134
APPARATUS 137
T-MAZE TEST 137
Requirements 138
Procedure 138
Observation 138
Applications for T-maze Test 139
Y-MAZE TEST 139
Requirements 140
Procedure 140
Observation 140
How is it different from T-maze? 141
Pros and cons of Y-maze over T-maze 142
Pros 142
Cons 142
NOVEL TANK TEST 143
Requirements 143

Procedure 143
Observation 144
Applications for Novel Tank Test 144
INHIBITORY AVOIDANCE TEST 145
Requirements 145
Procedure 145
Observation 146
Applications of Inhibitory Avoidance Test 146
LOCOMOTOR ACTIVITY TEST 147
Requirements 147
Procedure 147
Observation 148
Applications for Locomotor Activity Test 148
APPLICATIONS 148
ADVANTAGES OF LEARNING TESTS 149
LIMITATIONS OF LEARNING TESTS 150
PRACTICE QUESTIONS 150
REFERENCES 151

CHAPTER 19 NATIVE AREA RECOGNITION TEST IN ZEBRAFISH 152
Pratyush Porel, Falguni Goel and *Shamsher Singh*
INTRODUCTION 152
NATIVE AREA RECOGNITION TEST APPARATUS 152
Features of the Apparatus 154
ANY-maze Software 154
REQUIREMENTS 154
PROCEDURE 154
Preparation of the Setup 154
Testing Procedure 155
Data Analysis 155
Evaluation Criteria Duration in Every Zone 155
OBSERVATION 156
Graphical Presentation of Observation Table 157
RESULT 157
APPLICATIONS OF NATIVE AREA RECOGNITION TEST IN DISEASE OUTCOMES 157
ADVANTAGES 158
LIMITATIONS 159
PRACTICE QUESTIONS 159
REFERENCES 159

CHAPTER 20 VISUAL IMPAIRMENT TESTING IN ZEBRAFISH USING ROTATION TEST APPARATUS 161
Kousik Maparu and *Shamsher Singh*
INTRODUCTION 161
Features of the Apparatus 162
Instrument Specifications 162
REQUIREMENTS 162
PROCEDURE AND EVALUATION 163
Evaluation Method for Control Zebrafish 163
Evaluation of Mutant Zebrafish 163
OBSERVATION 164
Graphical Presentation of Observation Table 164

RESULT 164

APPLICATION 164

ADVANTAGES 165

LIMITATIONS 165

PRACTICE QUESTIONS 165

REFERENCES 165

CONCLUSION 166

BIBLIOGRAPHY 167

SUBJECT INDEX 172

FOREWORD

The Zebrafish has emerged as an indispensable model organism for advancing experimental pharmacology, offering unique insights into human disease and drug discovery. This handbook, *Zebrafish Models for Experimental Pharmacology*, aims to provide researchers, scientists, and pharmacologists with a comprehensive guide to utilizing Zebrafish in their experimental studies.

Covering the latest methodologies, experimental setups, and translational applications, the book delves into the versatility and biological relevance of Zebrafish for evaluating pharmacological agents and studying disease mechanisms. By compiling cutting-edge techniques and best practices, this handbook aspires to bridge the gap between foundational research and clinical application, empowering readers to harness the full potential of Zebrafish in innovative pharmacological research.

I have thoroughly reviewed the content and am pleased to forward this book, which I believe will be highly valuable to the scientific research community.

Y.K. Gupta
Pharmacology President, AIIMS
Bhopal, India

PREFACE

The goal of this book is to give readers a basic understanding of the subject's practical components, from handling Zebrafish and mounting tissue to the practical effects of several significant and intricate experimental techniques.

These days, experimental pharmacology has greatly strayed from the traditional method to focus on molecular and biochemical issues. Experimental pharmacology has been enhanced and expanded by advances in the fields of electrophysiology, biochemistry, molecular biology, electronic or digital recording methods, and software. Owing to the government's strict rules (CPCSEA), obtaining animals for research is a difficult undertaking.

Zebrafish have gained popularity as a model organism in biomedical research. Recently, researchers have been trying to better understand and cure conditions including cancer and various genetic and neurological abnormalities. One of Zebrafish's many benefits is that its embryo is transparent, making it possible to see how its tissues and organs grow and perform morphogenesis. This is crucial to comprehending the many systems that underlie health issues.

Some helpful elements of this book are available to the reader, such as the numerous worked-out examples that aid in putting theory into practice. A genuine effort was made to provide this book with as much pertinent material as possible, supporting it with appropriate examples and illustrated arguments. The subjects included in this book are carefully chosen in accordance with the majority of the contrived difficulties and the pharmacology curriculum. I believe this book will be useful to all recent graduates and postgraduates in the field of pharmacology, as well as to trainees and research personnel in their daily duties in allied health fields and toscientists in CROs with industrial drug development setups.

Several contemporary and straightforward experimental designs have been included to assist the students in their future drug discovery endeavors. Aside from this, the book covers a number of significant topics, including the ethics of using animals in experiments, how to handle and care for experimental animals, how to prepare solutions, and how to mount tissue for in vitro research.

Shamsher Singh
Neuropharmacology Division
Department of Pharmacology
ISF College of Pharmacy
Moga, Punjab 142001, India

Introduction

Zebrafish (*Danio rerio*) have emerged as a cornerstone of recent biomedical research, bridging the gap between genetic studies and developmental biology. Their unique attributes—transparent embryos, rapid development, capability for regeneration, and genetic manipulability—make them an ideal model organism for exploring complex biological processes and diseases. This handbook serves as a comprehensive resource, providing foundational knowledge and practical methodologies to enhance the understanding and application of Zebrafish across various scientific disciplines. The Zebrafish model offers several advantages over mammalian models, such as cost-effectiveness, high fecundity, and external fertilization, which allow real-time observation of development. Its genetic similarity to humans (approximately 70%) and rapid life cycle make it ideal for large-scale studies. Compared to mammalian models, Zebrafish also enable efficient genetic manipulations and drug screenings, significantly accelerating biomedical research.

The first chapter of the handbook offers a detailed overview of Zebrafish anatomy, lifecycle, and care requirements, crucial for creating optimal conditions for their growth and experimentation. It highlights the rapid development of embryos, which undergo significant transformations within the first 72 hours post-fertilization, leading to the formation of major organs. Additionally, the chapter emphasizes the importance of maintaining suitable environmental conditions, such as water quality and temperature, to ensure the fish's health. The second chapter examines various drug administration routes, including oral, intraperitoneal, and water-based methods, focusing on critical factors like dosage, timing, and absorption rates that affect experimental outcomes. Following this, blood collection techniques essential for biochemical and genetic analyses are discussed, detailing methods such as caudal vein and cardiac puncture, while underscoring ethical considerations to minimize discomfort and ensure humane treatment.

Anaesthesia is essential for procedures that may induce pain or distress in Zebrafish. The fourth chapter details commonly used anesthetic agents, their dosages, and their physiological effects, enabling researchers to anesthetize fish safely while prioritizing their welfare. Additionally, the book emphasizes the importance of Zebrafish as models for studying human diseases, supporting drug discovery and insights into disease mechanisms through genetic manipulation.

A substantial portion of the book is dedicated to various behavioural assays that enable researchers to explore cognitive and emotional responses in Zebrafish including shoaling behavior that reveals social dynamics and environmental influences, while the Novel Diving Tank Test (NDTT) assesses anxiety responses in unfamiliar settings. The Social Preference Test evaluates social interactions, and the Mirror Chamber Test investigates self-recognition and social cognition. The Three Chamber Test measures sociability, whereas the Light-Dark Chamber Test and Plus-Maze Test gauge anxiety levels by examining preferences for safe versus open environments. Spatial learning is assessed through the Y-Maze Test, Square-Maze Test, and T-Maze Test, which explore navigation and memory. The Novel Object Recognition Test (NORT) provides insights into cognitive function, while the Open Field Test measures general locomotion and exploration. The Learning Test evaluates task acquisition and retention, the Native Area Recognition Test assesses spatial memory, and the Zebrafish Rotation Test investigates motor coordination. Whether you are a seasoned researcher or a novice in the field, you will find valuable information that can enhance your research outcomes and inspire innovative applications.

As we navigate the intricate landscape of Zebrafish research, this handbook serves as your companion, equipping you with essential knowledge and practical techniques. By exploring the diverse applications of Zebrafish in experimental biology, we aim to inspire innovative research that advances our understanding of fundamental biological processes. Whether you are embarking on your first experiments or refining advanced methodologies, the insights and protocols contained within these pages will empower you to unlock the potential of this remarkable model organism. Together, let's dive into the fascinating world of Zebrafish and its contributions to science.

Shamsher Singh
Neuropharmacology Division
Department of Pharmacology
ISF College of Pharmacy
Moga, Punjab 142001, India

List of Contributors

Anupam Awasthi	Neuropharmacology Division, Department of Pharmacology, ISF College of Pharmacy, Moga, Punjab 142001, India
Dhrita Chatterjee	Neuropharmacology Division, Department of Pharmacology, ISF College of Pharmacy, Moga, Punjab 142001, India
Dilpreet Kaur	Neuropharmacology Division, Department of Pharmacology, ISF College of Pharmacy, Moga, Punjab 142001, India
Falguni Goel	Neuropharmacology Division, Department of Pharmacology, ISF College of Pharmacy, Moga, Punjab 142001, India
Kousik Maparu	Neuropharmacology Division, Department of Pharmacology, ISF College of Pharmacy, Moga, Punjab 142001, India
Khadga Raj	Neuropharmacology Division, Department of Pharmacology, ISF College of Pharmacy, Moga, Punjab 142001, India
Lav Goyal	Neuropharmacology Division, Department of Pharmacology, ISF College of Pharmacy, Moga, Punjab 142001, India
Lovekesh Singh	Neuropharmacology Division, Department of Pharmacology, ISF College of Pharmacy, Moga, Punjab 142001, India
Mayank Attri	Neuropharmacology Division, Department of Pharmacology, ISF College of Pharmacy, Moga, Punjab 142001, India
Nileshwar Kalia	Neuropharmacology Division, Department of Pharmacology, ISF College of Pharmacy, Moga, Punjab 142001, India
Pratyush Porel	Neuropharmacology Division, Department of Pharmacology, ISF College of Pharmacy, Moga, Punjab 142001, India
Omkar Kumar Kuwar	Neuropharmacology Division, Department of Pharmacology, ISF College of Pharmacy, Moga, Punjab 142001, India
Romanpreet Kaur	Neuropharmacology Division, Department of Pharmacology, ISF College of Pharmacy, Moga, Punjab 142001, India
Shamsher Singh	Neuropharmacology Division, Department of Pharmacology, ISF College of Pharmacy, Moga, Punjab 142001, India
Sania Grover	Neuropharmacology Division, Department of Pharmacology, ISF College of Pharmacy, Moga, Punjab 142001, India
Vaishali	Neuropharmacology Division, Department of Pharmacology, ISF College of Pharmacy, Moga, Punjab 142001, India

CHAPTER 1

Introduction and Basics to Zebrafish

Omkar Kumar Kuwar[1]**, Kousik Maparu**[1] **and Shamsher Singh**[1,*]

[1] *Neuropharmacology Division, Department of Pharmacology, ISF College of Pharmacy, Moga, Punjab 142001, India*

INTRODUCTION

Zebrafish: Zebrafish (*Danio rerio*), a freshwater teleost formerly used as an experimental model from the past few decades, is found in lakes and rivers [1]. They belong to the Minnow family Cyprindiae of Cypriniformes, native to South Asia [2]. Zebrafish derived its name from the five prominent, uniformly pigmented horizontal stripes that adorn its body, evoking the pattern of zebra-like stripes that cxtcnd longitudinally from the caudal fin and are distinctive characteristics of the species [3]. Zebrafish exhibit a fusiform (spindle-shaped) body plane, with lateral compression and a superiorly directed mouth, adapted for surface feeding and optimal maneuverability in its aquatic environment. Often referred to as tropical fish, this well-known aquarium fish is regularly offered for sale under the trade name Zebra Danio, also located in ponds. Female Zebrafish have silver stripes instead of gold and a wider white belly than males, a blue stripe separated by gold stripes in a torpedo design [4]. It takes three months to reach sexual maturity at 28.5°C and are considered adults in an ideal environment, Zebrafish commonly survive for 3-5 years [5, 6].

Nowadays, Zebrafish have evolved as a novel research model in recent decades as the species has many benefits such as being inexpensive to purchase, easy to maintain, handle, and breeding in the common laboratory. They are incredibly robust creatures. A single Zebrafish often yields between 20 and 200 offspring per breeding event. Other key advantages include: they are transparent during early developmental stages and have rapid development ability. Specifically, Zebrafish embryos develop from a single cell to a larva with a formed head, tail, and beating heart within 24 hours. In between 72 hours, the central nervous system is fully developed and becomes functional, and the fins become motile. By 5 days post-fertilization (dpf), they achieve full viability and are capable of independent swimming and foraging [7]. This rapid development and high reproductive output

---

* **Corresponding author Shamsher Singh:** Neuropharmacology Division, Department of Pharmacology, ISF College of Pharmacy, Moga, Punjab 142001, India; Tel: +91-9779980588; E-mail: shamshersinghbajwa@gmail.com

make Zebrafish an ideal model organism for both genetic and developmental biology research, particularly in high-throughput genetic studies. The basic organ system of Zebrafish is represented in Fig. (**1.1**).

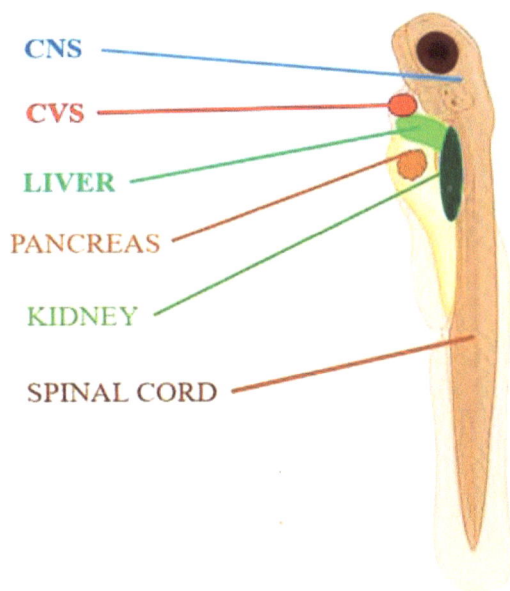

Fig. (1.1). Vital organs of Zebrafish.

ZEBRAFISH MAINTENANCE

As they are considered aquatic animals, they require good maintenance and care as per CPCSEA guidelines [8]. Various types of rotating systems constantly filter and oxygenate the water in which Zebrafish are kept to provide a marine environment that is favourable for their well-being. Fish waste products and extra foods are also filtered by the drainage system. Typically, the water and room temperature are kept between 26-28.5 °C and 12 hr light: 12 hr dark cycle. Un-purified water is passed through another tank after passing through a UV disinfection filter followed by a biological and active carbon absorption filter, a 50-micron canister filter, and finally 120-micron filter pad. To make dechlorinated water, it should be kept for at least 48 hours in a chamber and water should be circulated by a pump to keep it warm and speed up the dechlorination process [9].

The water pH-controller system should be monitored every day and pH should be kept around 6.8 to 7.5. $NaHCO_3$ can be used to raise pH levels while required. It is important to clean fish tanks regularly. While cleaning the tank, stop the water supply and tilt the tank back to release the remaining water, and then carefully remove the tank from the system. Dirt accumulation and the growth of algae/fungus may be observed at the side walls and bottom of the tank. After filling the tank with dechlorinated water, place the baffle inside a clean tank. Using a fish net, carefully transfer fish into the tank and then shut the cover. Slide the cleaned tank into the system gently, then turn on the water supply. Before reusing the net, spray it with seventy percent ethanol, again rinse it with water, and allow it to dry. Take off the baffle from the unclean tank then spray with the same on both sides. Before reusing, give the tank and baffles a thorough rinse under tap water and let them completely dry. The filters need to be routinely checked and replaced with the circulation system to operate properly. Ensure that the water supply in each fish tank is neat and clean and that the filters are replaced regularly. Before replacing the 120-micron filter pad, make sure to reposition the filter toward the direction of water flow and utilize it completely before replacing it with a new one. Every week, the canister filter needs to be replaced. Use a wrench or your hands to spin the filter unit anticlockwise to remove it and then replace the canister filter and place a towel underneath to avoid or absorb water spills. Following the replacement of the old canister filter with a new one, carefully reinstall the filter into the aquatic system, manually adjusting its position as necessary. Twice every week or once every two weeks, the carbon filter needs to be replaced [10].

Use a wrench to carefully remove the carbon filter unit to replace the carbon filter. Replace the used activated carbon with fresh carbon by discarding it. Place the carbon holder back into the filter unit after re-fitting it. Reinstall the filtration unit inside the system. Before putting the filter into the system, flush some water through the pipes to clear all extra particles. Every six months, the biological filter needs to be washed. In a circulating system, a biological filter is often positioned between the carbon filter and the canister. Press the button for pressure release to reduce the filter pressure. For this phase, two people are usually required. After removing the filter's lid, extract the spore from the water and empty the contents of the filter into a container with a sieve. Nitrification and de-nitrification are two processes where a fine-pore bio-filter medium is used to separate spores [10].

Restore the spores in a fresh tank if the previous one is not clear. Replace the filter unit's lid, add de-chlorinated water, put it back into the system, and then turn on the water supply. Several nitrifying bacteria will reside in the spore in an acclimated aquarium. Because the nitrogen cycle in the aquarium depends on these microorganisms, remove the dirty spore which could cause a significant rise in ammonia (NH_3) and nitrite ($N \equiv C-$) as compared to the new biological filter, which contains the clean spores. If it is not handled properly, either of these nitrogen cycle intermediate stages may be hazardous to aquatic life and even fatal to Zebrafish. Consequently, the Zebrafish housing system needs another biological filter somewhere to facilitate the quick repopulation of crucial microorganisms on the new spores. UV filters should be changed every nine to ten months to control biological impurities (like bacteria) in the system. It should be mentioned that even though the globe seems to be in good working order, it is important to replace it since the UV filter disinfection dosage rate is 110 mill joules per square centimeter at the start of the bulb life then drops with time [9, 10].

FEEDING

Zebrafish should be provide a balanced diet by combining dry and live feeds. Food size varies from 100µ in the case of larvae and for adults 300-400µ in diameter, brine shrimp. The preferred salinity range for culturing brine shrimp is 35-40 ppt (specific gravity 1.024-1.028). The following procedures are outlined below that can be used to produce brine shrimp (Artemia sp.) eggs:

1. Red sea salt is dissolved in water in a beaker and set on a magnetic stirrer to increase dispersion. Alternatively, you might oxygenate the water and mix the mineral salt in it using the airflow hose pipe. If red sea salt is unavailable, then use instant marine salt as a hatching medium. We hatch the brine shrimp (12–15g) in red sea salt water with 30-35 g/L of salt, even though brine shrimps can cope with a wide range of salinities (<1%) as well in brine shrimp eggs are difficult to obtain at local pet stores, enclosed brine shrimp may be used instead, provided they are "decapped" in smaller batches before being introduced into the shrimp hatchery [10].
2. Before putting shrimp eggs into the brine shrimp hatcher, add 1-2 teaspoons of saltwater per liter. Use a pump to provide the hatcher a good ventilation and enable shrimp to hatch eggs in about 48 hours. It is important to note that unenriched shrimp brine loses its nutritional value rapidly after hatching. It is advisable to either extend hatching over 24 hours or enrich them over 48 hours to maximize their nutritional content [9, 10].
3. Before wastewater was combined with contaminated waste, it is treated with chlorine in an incubator.

To facilitate brine shrimp collection, disconnect the air hose and allow the culture to settle for 3 to 5 minutes, ensuring not to exceed 10 minutes of brine shrimp aggregate near the bottom inside the hatcher [9, 10].

1. Use a tap, located at the bottom of the hatching place, gather brine shrimp, and discard the first batch of eggs where brine shrimp had not yet hatched.
2. Also, discard the unhatched brine shrimp and collect the originated ones that will be provided to Zebrafish.

3. Retrieve brine shrimp from salted water using a brine shrimp collection net made of approximately 350-micron nylon screen. By using water from the system, wash brine shrimp from the net into a dish.

The bottom of the container usually has a large concentration of the gathered brine shrimp which gives it an orange hue. When food is added to the water, fish dive to grab the brine shrimp. A pipette, dropper, and squeezy bottle are used to feed the brine shrimp. The amount of food delivered to the tank is determined by the population of fish in the tank. For Zebrafish, the recommended daily feeding ratio is 3–4% of their body weight. Overfeeding should not be done as this can raise the nitrate level in the water and perhaps harm the reproductive ability and rate of survival of Zebrafish may even die from overeating [9, 10].

A basic spring-based fish food dispenser seen in Aquatic Eco-Systems (Aquatic habitats) can be used for dry feeding. An alternative for dry feeding is to use a regular spoon or cut a plastic dropper in half diagonally [9].

To attain superior testing results and maintain a healthy diet, food specifically designed for Zebrafish is recommended. As the fish mature, feeding is done based on their age and typically occurs 2-3 times a day. Depending on the nature of the experiment conducted, the fish larvae may benefit from more frequent feeding [9 - 11].

BREEDING

Breeding in zebrafish refers to the process of facilitating reproduction in Zebrafish.

1. Identify male and female fishes and transfer them into the mating tanks, which are separated by a transparent divider. The larger underbelly of females helps to identify them from males because they are darker in color and slenderer than females on the other hand, male fishes can also be easily identified as females. In addition, male's anal fins are more yellow-colored than females. If any doubt arises, check female Zebrafish for the ovipositor [9 - 11].
2. Keep the mating tank undisturbed overnight in the dark. When light begins to appear in the morning, remove the divider. Give 20 minutes to complete mating or until enough embryos have dropped to the bottom of the tank.
3. In-tank paired breeding can provide fertile eggs. In-tank mating can be a more labour-efficient method for collecting embryos in the lab while paired mating is recommended for examining genetics or polymorphisms within specific species.
4. Collect the fertilized eggs and transfer the fish to another tank once they have laid eggs in the breeding tank.

5. Reintroduce the species into their tanks after breeding. Transfer the larvae to another cleaned dish. Use sterilized water to completely wash the embryos. Wash the mesh screen with a specific embryo medium (EM3), before transferring the embryos to a Petri plate, (EM3) composed of the following ionic components (Table **1.1**).

Subsequently, we examine the embryos under a microscope. Utilize a Pasteur pipette to separate fertilized eggs from unfertilized ones.

Table 1.1. Ionic components of specific embryo medium [9].

S. No.	Components	Quantity
1.	Disodium phosphate	0.025 mM
2.	Monopotassium phosphate	0.044 mM
3.	Sodium bicarbonate	4.2 mM
4.	Potassium chloride	0.54 mM
5.	Calcium chloride	1.3 mM
6.	Sodium chloride	13.7 mM
7.	Magnesium sulfate	1.0 mM

Caring of Larvae

1. The fertilized embryos are kept in an incubation chamber (28.5°C) for 72–80 hours until embryos leave the embryonic sac. Now that the juveniles are free to swim outside of the chorion, they are ready to be transferred to a large fish aquarium. Larvae can be maintained in circular dishes with daily water changes. Along with any other debris, dead or unhealthy larvae should be removed during the water change.
2. Gently place the larvae inside the tank with a tiny baffle (about 300–400 microns). A few millilitres of water should be gradually added every day and if any dead or sick larvae are found they should be removed.
3. Larvae tanks might be added to the circulatory system after 14 days and a tiny trickle of cycling water (1 or 2 drops/second) can be provided. The flow of water can be accelerated once the larvae develop. Concerning the size or age of the larvae, a variety of baffle lengths (300–350, 400–500, 700–750, and 900–1000 microns) can be utilized; for adult fish, a regular plastic baffle can be used [9 - 11].
4. It generally takes 90 days for the embryos to become sexually mature adults, in an ideal condition [5].

ZEBRAFISH AS A MODEL

George Streisinger and collaborators at the University of Oregon proposed using Zebrafish (*Danio rerio*) as a biomedical model because they are superior to other species in numerous ways, the benefits of using Zebrafish as a model are external fertilization and less development time from embryo to adult around 3 months, fast embryonic development of fewer than 24 hours, well-sequenced genome, simple genome manipulation, and high fecundity. After 48 hours-post-fertilization (hpf), embryos grow into whole organ systems, including gut, heart, and blood vessels [12]. In scientific research, Zebrafish are a valuable and frequently utilized model organism of vertebrates as they share many similarities with the mammalian brain, including the rat brain, in terms of structure, function, and genetic pathways. The similarity between Zebrafish and mouse brains is shown in Fig. (**1.2**); these similarities make zebrafish an excellent model for studying neurological processes and diseases, as they allow for high-throughput screening and genetic manipulation, providing insights that are often translatable to mammalian systems.

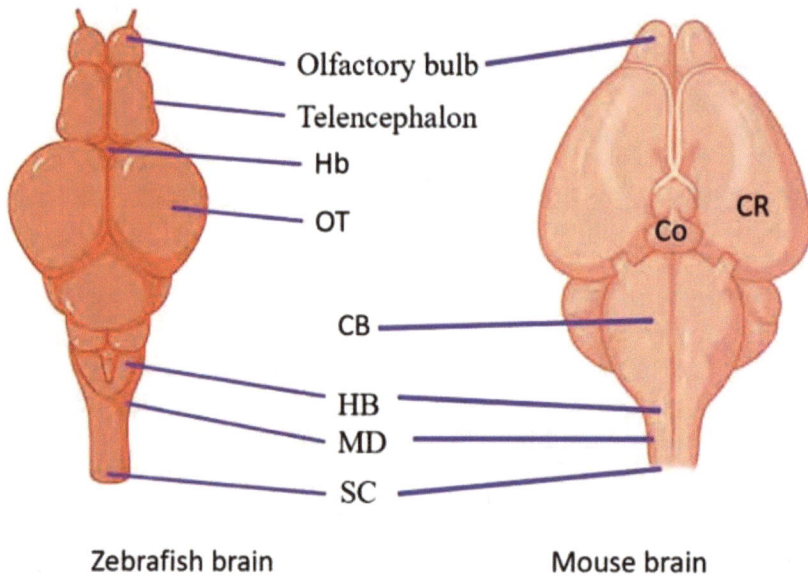

Fig. (1.2). A comprehensive diagram of Zebrafish & Mouse brain. SC - spinal cord, OT - optic tectum, CB - cerebellum, MD - medulla, Hb - habenula, CR - cortex, HB - hindbrain, Co –colliculi.

Developmental biology and biomedicine have utilized Zebrafish. Zebrafish is an alternative animal model which follows 3R approaches (Fig. **1.3**) [13].

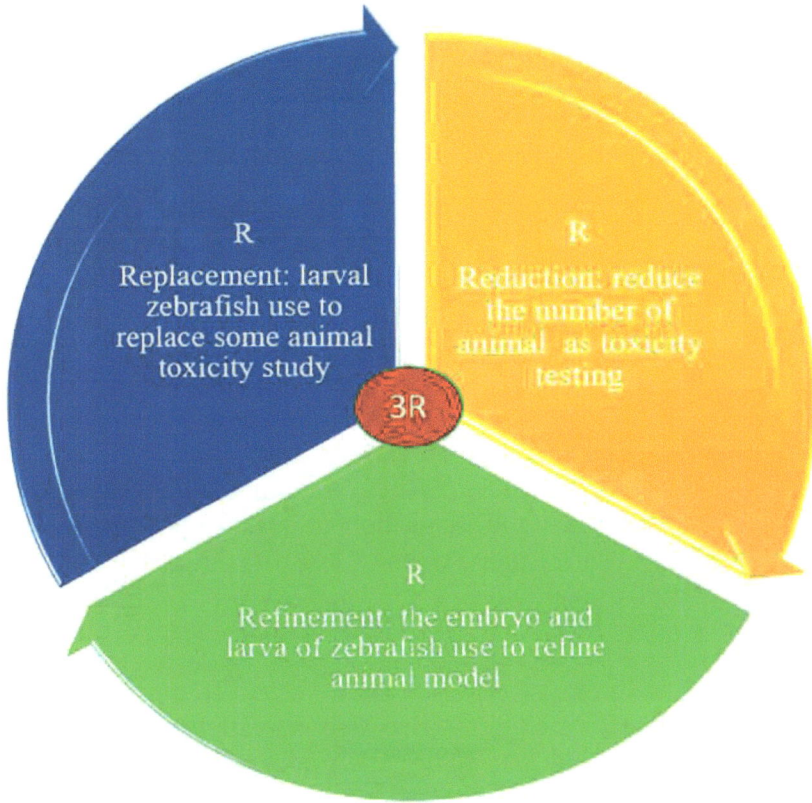

Fig. (1.3). 3R approaches of Zebrafish using as a model.

It may be surprising to know that, despite our apparent differences, humans and Zebrafish share a great deal of similarities. Indeed, Zebrafish contain 70% similarity of human genes. The heart, ear, pancreas, liver, bile passages, bone, cartilage kidneys, stomach, nose, muscle, blood, and teeth are among the anatomical features of Zebrafish. They also have two sets of eyes, a brain, a vertebral column, and a digestive tract. Humans as well as Zebrafish share multiple genes, and the essential pathways required to develop these traits. As a result, Zebrafish can potentially mimic any condition of humans that modifies several physiological components.

Zebrafish are also used for different types of *in-vivo* and *in-vitro* assays including Zebrafish embryo toxicity assay, behavioral toxicity assay, and cytotoxicity assays in Zebrafish cell lines [14].

Thus, detailed organ analysis makes use of Zebrafish. The species is used for the following studies:

Toxicity Analysis

Zebrafish are extensively used to investigate the etiology and origins of neurological conditions and disorders for toxicity study and drug discovery process. The larvae of Zebrafish deliver more accurate data for toxicity study.

Ocular Toxicity

Zebrafish and human eyes possess various similar anatomical features such as the retina, choroid, cornea, vascularization, lens, and innervation and also share similar structures and organization of tissues, gene regulation, and cellular composition. That's why Zebrafish is considered an outstanding model to study ocular toxicity. Optical stimulation such as vision is developed in Zebrafish after 5 dpf. Environmental exposure such as various drugs, heavy metals, cosmetics, care products, chemicals, retardants, plastics, and agrochemicals showed adverse effects on Zebrafish embryos and disruption in visual performance. Oxidative stress, agrochemicals, and polystyrene are responsible for producing inflammatory markers including IL-4, IL-1β, CXCL, CLC, IL-8, and TNF-α responsible for ocular toxicity. Zebrafish's visual system consists of the extraocular muscles, optic nerve, neural retina, and optic tectum [15].

Optokinetic and optomotor are mainly two assays available to analyze adult and larval Zebrafish's vision, and also light-dark preference test, phototaxis, visual avoidance behavior analysis, and free-swimming activity used to analyze visual performance described in Table **1.2.**

Table 1.2. Various testing assay procedures for checking ocular toxicity and apparatus.

S. No.	Visual Testing Procedures	Apparatus
01.	Optokinetic assay	

(Table 1.2) cont.....

S. No.	Visual Testing Procedures	Apparatus
02.	Optomotor assay	
03.	Light–dark preference test	
04.	Visual avoidance behavior analysis	
05.	Phototaxis	

Neurotoxicity

Zebrafish contain more than 26,000 protein-coding genes and 26 pairs of chromosomes and show about 70% homology with the human genome. Zebrafish is extensively used for various neurological manifestations and disorders.

Photo-motor response assay is performed to determine the locomotor activity, a light-dark assay is used for a depressive-like neurological disorder and a touch-evoked response test depicts tactile stimulus performed in Zebrafish. Various toxins such as MPTP cause neurobehavioral toxicity in dopaminergic neurons in Zebrafish. For neurotoxicity analysis various instruments are used to determine behavioral changes, some of the instruments are represented in Fig. (**1.4**).

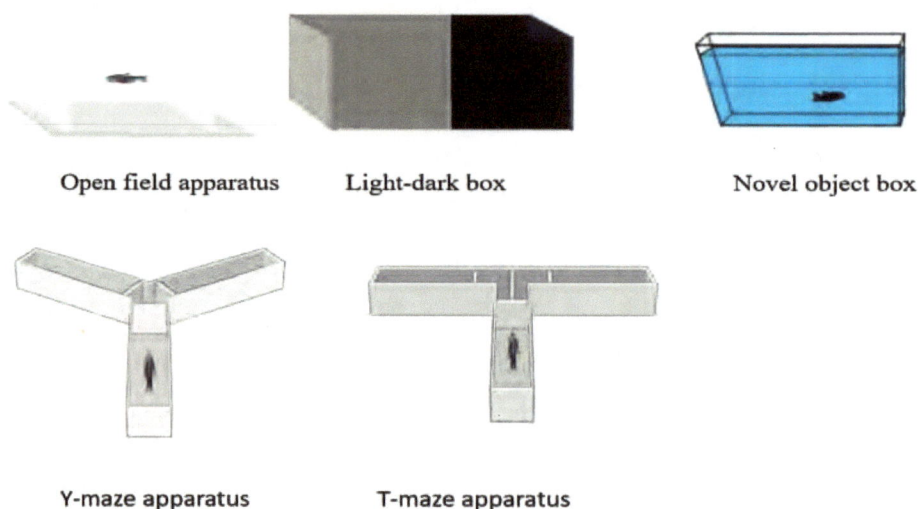

Open field apparatus   Light-dark box   Novel object box

Y-maze apparatus   T-maze apparatus

Fig. (1.4). Various testing apparatuses used in Zebrafish determine various parameters of behavioral changes in toxicity study [16].

Embryotoxicity

According to OECD 236 guidelines, a validated procedure of acute toxicity test for fish embryos is well established. Different types of chemical exposure cause toxicity in Zebrafish embryos if a new fertilized egg is exposed for about 96 hours and shows different morphological disabilities in the embryo, including;

• Disorganize or absent somite
• Coagulation of eggs
• Improper heart formation, and pericardial oedema

- Developing oedema or swelling area of the yolk-sac and detachment of the yolk-sac from the tail bud

From this type of morphological end-point evaluation, we can determine the toxicity of any drug or chemical using Zebrafish embryos.

Cardiovascular Toxicity

Zebrafish are an excellent model for determining cardiotoxicity as they have conserved cellular and anatomical similarities to humans. They can regenerate their heart muscle, so studies are going on to investigate the factors or methods involved in this ability for regeneration. Different types of assay are performed in Zebrafish for toxicity testing, such as high throughput screening assay for bradycardia in Zebrafish embryos [17].

Toxicity in other organs

Pancreas

Zebrafish is used for pancreatic research to investigate the endocrine segment and evaluate islets' protection and damage but does not focus on polypeptide-producing cells because it is not identified in Zebrafish. Chemical toxicity of the exocrine pancreas is focused on the embryo developmental model.

Intestine

Zebrafish model is extensively used for various intestinal disorders for investigation of the microbiome, intestinal inflammation, and congenital disorder but there are some limitations found regarding the absence of path cells, crypt cells, and payer's patches in the intestine of Zebrafish.

Liver

Zebrafish liver starts its full function after 5dpf and shows the same function as humans although liver cells of Zebrafish are less organized but present all the same types of cells as mammals. Different fluorescent markers (Resazurin) are used to determine real changes in Zebrafish liver for toxicity testing of any chemical.

Benefits of using Zebrafish as a Model

To emphasize the advantages of the Zebrafish model, it is indeed valuable to compare it with similar mammalian models. Following the introduction of the Zebrafish model, such comparisons can highlight its unique benefits, such as cost-effectiveness, high-throughput capabilities, and ease of genetic manipulation, alongside its limitations, such as reduced physiological complexity compared to mammals. This approach provides a balanced perspective, showcasing how Zebrafish complement mammalian models in experimental research.

1. They are small and easy to handle.
2. Their genome is about 70% like humans.
3. Cheaper to maintain than other laboratory animals such as mice, rats, and rabbits.
4. Zebrafish embryos are almost transparent, so scientists may easily study how internal structures grow.

Limitations of using Zebrafish as a Model

1. Due to having some dissimilarities in respiratory and reproductive systems, this type of study may be difficult to perform.
2. Many genes are present in two copies so determining the functional role of a particular gene becomes difficult.
3. Physiology is not the same as humans.

Application of Zebrafish as an Experimental Model

Zebrafish are a great model for ecotoxicological investigations, neurological studies, and metabolic problems. They are especially suitable for embryonic studies due to their remarkably translucent body throughout the larval development. Zebrafish display similar biological processes due to their similar physiological characteristics and genetic makeup, which makes them model organisms in many cases. Utilizing fluorescent reporters or tagged proteins in Zebrafish, CRISPR-Cas9 genome editing techniques are used to create disease models and investigate mechanisms of action for a variety of investigations.

Zebrafish provide a superior model for studying human disease than other vertebrates, particularly when it comes to screening large genetic mutations, assessing therapeutic compounds, and conducting a large variety of biomedical experiments [18]. Various applications of Zebrafish as a research model are represented in Fig. (**1.5**).

PRACTICE QUESTIONS

1. Discuss briefly about Zebrafish maintenance and care.
2. Describe the details of the Zebrafish feeding procedure.
3. What are the applications of Zebrafish as an experimental model?
4. What type of toxicity testing is performed in Zebrafish?
5. Discuss the breeding procedures of Zebrafish.

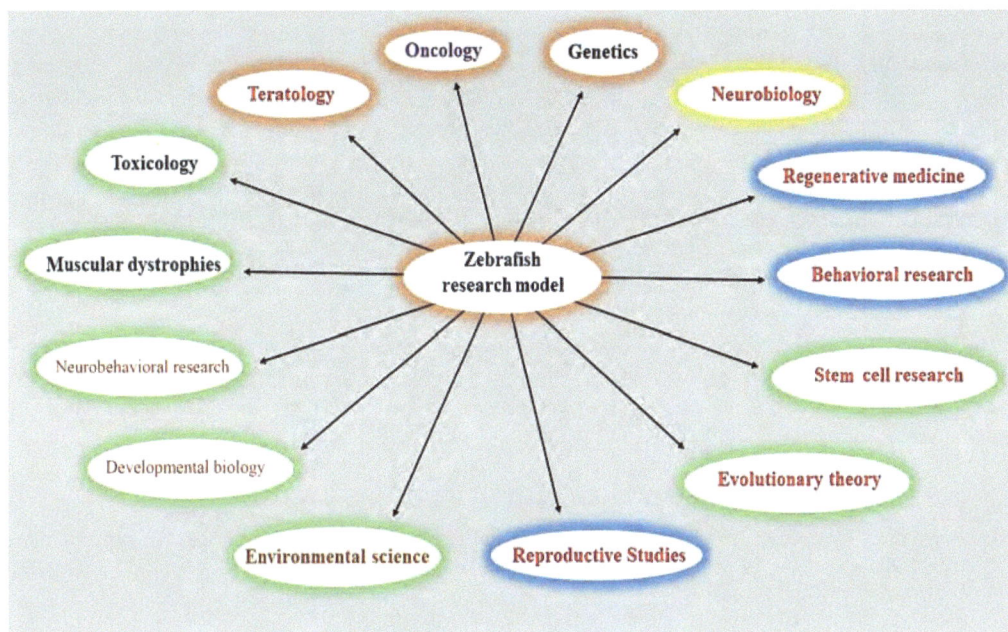

Fig. (1.5). Various applications of Zebrafish as a research model.

REFERENCES

[1]   Khan FR, Alhewairini S. Zebrafish (*Danio rerio*) as a model organism. Curr Trends Cancer Manag 2018; 27: 3-18.

[2]   Teame T, Zhang Z, Ran C, *et al.* The use of zebrafish (*Danio rerio*) as biomedical models. Anim Front 2019; 9(3): 68-77.
[http://dx.doi.org/10.1093/af/vfz020] [PMID: 32002264]

[3]   JoVE Science Education. 2023.

[4]   Sharma M. Perspective on zebrafish: a suitable research model. J Exp Zool India 2012; 15(2): 303-7.

[5]   Maqsood HM, Jaias I, Mattoo AI, Akram T, Akram W, Ganai NA. Breeding of zebrafish and its life cycle. In: Zebrafish as a model for Parkinson's disease. CRC Press 2024; 29-42.
[http://dx.doi.org/10.1201/9781003402893-4]

[6]   Gerhard GS, Kauffman EJ, Wang X, *et al.* Life spans and senescent phenotypes in two strains of Zebrafish (*Danio rerio*). Exp Gerontol 2002; 37(8-9): 1055-68.
[http://dx.doi.org/10.1016/S0531-5565(02)00088-8] [PMID: 12213556]

[7]   Fraysse B, Mons R, Garric J. Development of a zebrafish 4-day embryo-larval bioassay to assess toxicity of chemicals. Ecotoxicol Environ Saf 2006; 63(2): 253-67.
[http://dx.doi.org/10.1016/j.ecoenv.2004.10.015] [PMID: 16677909]

[8]   Patra S, Bala A, Sharma N, Haldar PK. Developmental toxicity assessment of *Drymaria cordata* (Linn.) Willd using zebrafish embryo. Curr Drug Saf 2023; 18(2): 214-23.
[http://dx.doi.org/10.2174/1574886317666220514153858] [PMID: 35570534]

[9]   Avdesh A, Chen M, Martin-Iverson MT, *et al.* Regular care and maintenance of a zebrafish (*Danio rerio*) laboratory: an introduction. J Vis Exp 2012; (69): e4196.
[PMID: 23183629]

[10] Aleström P, D'Angelo L, Midtlyng PJ, *et al.* Zebrafish: Housing and husbandry recommendations. Lab Anim 2020; 54(3): 213-24.
[http://dx.doi.org/10.1177/0023677219869037] [PMID: 31510859]

[11] Longkumer S, Jamir A, Pranay PP. Maintenance and breeding of zebrafish under laboratory conditions for animal research. Agric Sci Dig 2024; 44(3): 551-5.

[12] Verma SK, Nandi A, Sinha A, Patel P, Mohanty S, Jha E, *et al.* The posterity of Zebrafish in paradigm of *in vivo* molecular toxicological profiling. Biomed Pharmacother 2024; 171: 116160.
[http://dx.doi.org/10.1016/j.biopha.2024.116160]

[13] Bailone RL, Fukushima HCS, Fernandes BHV, *et al.* Zebrafish as an alternative animal model in human and animal vaccination research. Lab Anim Res 2020; 36(1): 13.
[http://dx.doi.org/10.1186/s42826-020-00042-4]

[14] Zhao W, Chen Y, Hu N, Long D, Cao Y. The uses of zebrafish (*Danio rerio*) as an *in vivo* model for toxicological studies: A review based on bibliometrics. Ecotoxicol Environ Saf 2024; 272: 116023.

[15] Yi J, Ma Y, Ma J, *et al.* Rapid assessment of ocular toxicity from environmental contaminants based on visually mediated zebrafish behavior studies. Toxics 2023; 11(8): 706.
[http://dx.doi.org/10.3390/toxics11080706] [PMID: 37624211]

[16] Benvenutti R, Marcon M, Gallas-Lopes M, de Mello AJ, Herrmann AP, Piato A. Swimming in the maze: An overview of maze apparatuses and protocols to assess zebrafish behavior. Neurosci Biobehav Rev 2021; 127: 761-78.
[http://dx.doi.org/10.1016/j.neubiorev.2021.05.027] [PMID: 34087275]

[17] Wei Y, Meng Y, Huang Y, *et al.* Development toxicity and cardiotoxicity in zebrafish from exposure to iprodione. Chemosphere 2021; 263: 127860.
[http://dx.doi.org/10.1016/j.chemosphere.2020.127860]

[18] Choi TY, Choi TI, Lee YR, Choe SK, Kim CH. Zebrafish as an animal model for biomedical research. Exp Mol Med 2021; 53(3): 310-7.
[http://dx.doi.org/10.1038/s12276-021-00571-5] [PMID: 33649498]

CHAPTER 2

Routes of Drug Administration in Zebrafish

Kousik Maparu[1] and **Shamsher Singh**[1,*]

[1] *Neuropharmacology Division, Department of Pharmacology, ISF College of Pharmacy, Moga, Punjab 142001, India*

INTRODUCTION

Aim: To study various methods of drug administration in Zebrafish.

Scope and Outcomes: This chapter covers a thorough about various routes of drug administration techniques for Zebrafish with the goal of clarifying the steps involved and the results that are necessary to progress biomedical research. This chapter will cover a variety of techniques, including intramuscular (*i.m.*), intraperitoneally (*i.p.*), and intrathoracic injections, and will offer thorough guidance on performing these procedures successfully. By following these detailed protocols, researchers will obtain more reproducible results in their studies involving Zebrafish.

Theory: Drug delivery involves introducing medicinal substances into the body to target specific cells *in vivo* for the treatment of various disorders. It encompasses two key components: dosage form and delivery route. Effective drug administration ensures optimal drug action by regulating drug release, cellular absorption, and proper distribution within the body. Common methods of drug administration include enteral (*via* the digestive system), parenteral (injections), inhalation (*via* the nasal passages), transdermal (through the skin), topical (applied to the skin), and oral (*via* the mouth) [1]. Choosing the appropriate delivery method is critical to maximizing therapeutic effects while minimizing toxicity, particularly when targeting specific organs such as the brain or utilizing advanced drug delivery systems. In Zebrafish, drug administration presents unique challenges due to their small size and aquatic habitat. Various techniques have been developed to deliver drug substances effectively for research purposes.

---

* **Corresponding author Shamsher Singh:** Neuropharmacology Division, Department of Pharmacology, ISF College of Pharmacy, Moga, Punjab 142001, India; Tel: +91-9779980588; E-mail: shamshersinghbajwa@gmail.com

Below are some key considerations for drug administration in Zebrafish [2]:

1. **Water-soluble substances:** It can be difficult to keep the medicine concentrations that the fish ingest constant when water-soluble substances are added straight to the water in the aquarium [3].
2. **Food-based medicine pellets:** Medicated food pellets are an effective method for administering medication to adult Zebrafish, particularly for long-term therapies. This technique ensures precise, consistent, and non-invasive dosing, making it both practical and less stressful for the fish [4].
3. **Injections and oral gavage:** Although these techniques provide accurate dosage control, they are intrusive, potentially hazardous, and necessitate anesthesia, particularly when administered repeatedly.
4. **Inserts for spawning:** Zebrafish can be exposed to medicine by being submerged in a solution through inserts for spawning, which allows for accurate dosage for multiple fish at once. Different ways of drug administration with examples of models are described in Table **2.1**.

Table 2.1. Various routes of drug administration along with examples.

S. No.	Different Techniques	Examples of Drugs that Generally Administered with Different Techniques
01	Bath immersion	Antiepileptic drugs, such as Zebrafish larvae exhibit seizure-like behaviors that mimic human epilepsy. Useful when administering hydrophilic drugs targeting the GI tract.
02	Microinjection	Delivery of neurotoxins or chemotherapeutic agents to evaluate their effects on behavior and physiology. Allows conduct of toxicity assessments for compounds.
03	Oral delivery	Micropipette and needle-based method. Metabolic and obesity studies.
04	Target drug delivery (Nanoparticles, Hydrogels, *etc.*)	Target-specific drug delivery. Real-time measurement of accumulation and distribution.

REQUIREMENTS

Animal: Adult Zebrafish

Equipment: Syringe, micro-needles, micropipette, micro-injection.

PROCEDURES

Intra-muscular (*i.m.*)

Drugs deliver into dorsal muscle in adult Zebrafish (Fig. **2.1**).

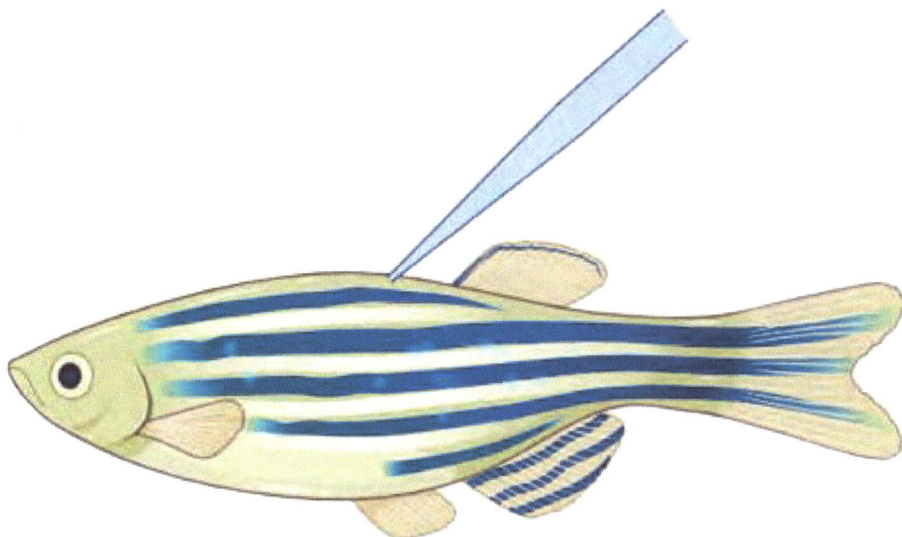

Fig. (2.1). Intra muscular (*i.m.*) in Zebrafish.

Preparation: Anesthetize the Zebrafish using tacrine, then position its dorsal side up on a moist sponge. Place the fish under a microscope and place a 45-degree angle micro-injection needle close to the dorsal muscle.

Injection: To put the needle, locate a scale-free location in front of the dorsal fin. Slowly inject phenol red and the desired ingredient (such as a DNA vaccination) into the muscle tissue after carefully inserting the needle.

Electroporation: If the chemical contains genetic material, use electrodes on both sides of the injection site to electroporate the region. Using an electroporator, deliver six pulses of 40 volts for 50 milliseconds each to help muscle cells absorb genetic material.

Recovery: After the procedure, move the fish right away to a recovery tank.

Monitoring: Use UV light to detect enhanced green fluorescent protein (EGFP) expression at the injection site as an indicator of successful uptake and expression of the genetic material.

Intra-peritoneal (*i.p.*)

Drugs are delivered into the abdominal cavity by *i.p.* route [5] (Fig. **2.2**).

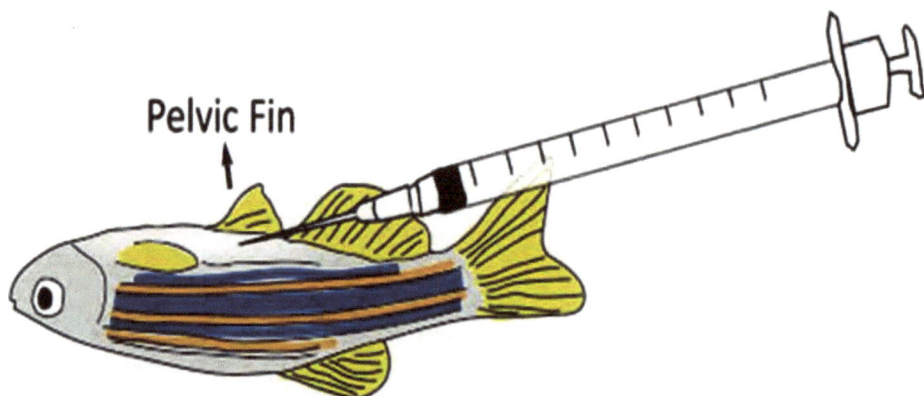

Fig. (2.2). Intraperitoneally (*i.p.*) injection in Zebrafish.

Preparation: The adult Zebrafish should fast for a full day before injection to empty its gastrointestinal tract and make space in its abdomen. Use tricaine to anesthetize the fish, then place its ventral side up in a slot on a wet sponge.

Injection procedure: The injection procedure involves pipetting the required amount of the injection solution onto laboratory film and then loading it onto a 30-gauge insulin needle. The needle should be inserted 45 degrees from the anterior-posterior body axis between the pelvic fins. Slowly inject the solution after gently inserting the needle 1 to 2 millimeters into the abdominal cavity.

Post-injection: To avoid spilling, wait five seconds after injecting the needle. Put the fish in a recovery tank with fresh tank water as soon as possible. If the fish does not start swimming right away after injection, aid in recovery by gently swirling water near the gills.

Monitoring and experiment: For this experiment, select adult Zebrafish aged five to eight months, including one wild-type fish and one RAG1 mutant fish. Monitor the fish regularly for any signs of infection throughout the study. Every 15 minutes, collect bacterial samples from the injected fluid and plate them on 7H10 agar. Incubate the plates at 29°C for five days to determine the infection dose. This procedure ensures accurate monitoring of bacterial growth and infection dynamics.

Health monitoring and euthanasia: Regularly check the well-being of the fish. Euthanize any fish showing infection symptoms by immersing them in water containing more than 0.02% of 3-aminobenzoic acid ethyl ester.

Intrathoracic

Drug delivery into the heart *via* intrathoracic cavity [6] (Fig. **2.3**).

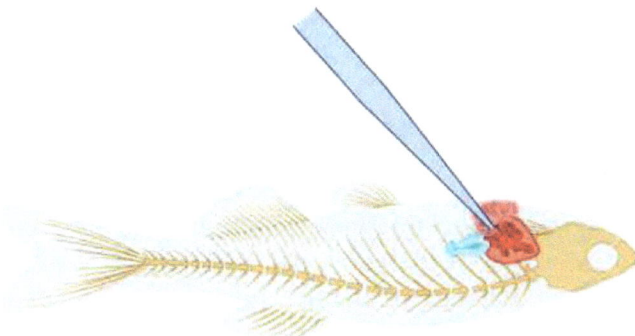

Fig. (2.3). Intrathoracic injection in Zebrafish.

Preparation: Place a wet sponge with a slit in a Petri dish. Apply tricaine to an adult Zebrafish to make it unconscious, then carefully place it with its ventral side facing up in the slit. To see the beating heart, place the Petri dish under a stereo microscope.

Procedure for Injection: A microinjection needle should be positioned between the operculum and the pectoral girdle, at a 45-degree angle above the beating heart. Gently insert the needle into the pericardium, the membrane that surrounds the heart, through the skin. To track the migration of the pericardium, inject the necessary solution (such as a test chemical with a tracer dye like phenol red). Different angles of a given injection in routes are described in Table **2.2**.

Post injection: Remove the needle from the thorax. Move the fish right away into a rehabilitation tank that has system water in it. Observe the fish until its anesthetic wears off completely.

Analysis: To analyze the effects of the injection, collect the heart at the desired time point. Get ready to analyze the cardiac tissue more thoroughly, perhaps through histology or molecular research.

Table 2.2. Angles of different routes of administering drugs in Zebrafish.

S. No.	Routes	Angle
1.	Intramuscular (*i.m.*)	45˚
2.	Intraperitoneally (*i.p.*) injection	45˚
3.	Intrathoracic injection	45˚

RESULT

Different routes of drug administration in Zebrafish were understood and performed successfully.

APPLICATIONS

1. **Disease modeling and pathophysiology:** Administering drugs or chemical compounds in Zebrafish can be effectively modeled through genetic manipulation. This approach allows scientists to study various diseases and monitor their progression and treatment in a controlled environment.
2. **Genetic and molecular studies:** Genetic material (DNA and RNA) can be examined to learn more about the regulatory systems, gene expression patterns, and mutations that affect the growth and function of blood cells.
3. **Assays:** By administering the drug, we perform various types of assays of any chemical compounds in Zebrafish.
4. **Drug discovery and toxicology:** Zebrafish are crucial for evaluating the efficacy and toxicity of pharmaceutical compounds. Researchers can assess how drugs affect Zebrafish.
5. **Targeted drug delivery system:** By different routes, we can target different organs for drug delivery.

ADVANTAGES

1. **Non-invasive:** Fish discomfort and stress can be minimized using non-invasive approaches such as spawning inserts and food-based medication pellets.
2. **Precise dosing:** The amount of medication given to each fish can be precisely controlled using these methods.
3. **Long-term treatments:** They work well for long-term medication regimens for spawning inserts, which are crucial for researching the impacts of repeated drug exposure.
4. **Relevance to mammalian models:** The Zebrafish model allows for versatile drug administration routes, including immersion, injection, and oral delivery, enabling rapid and cost-effective testing. Unlike mammalian models, Zebrafish embryos and larvae can absorb compounds directly through their permeable skin and gills, simplifying experimental procedures and reducing resource requirements.
5. **Monitor pharmacokinetics**: By various routes, we can monitor different pharmacokinetic properties in Zebrafish such as absorption, and distribution.

LIMITATIONS

1. **Water soluble compounds:** If water-soluble substances are added straight to

fish water, the fish may absorb drugs at unknown concentrations.

2. **Invasive methods**: Oral gavage and injection methods are invasive as well as sometimes fatal, which concerns animal welfare.

FUTURE DIRECTIONS

1. **Gene editing:** More accurate modeling of human diseases is possible by using gene editing methods like CRISPR-Cas9 to introduce certain mutations or gene knockouts in Zebrafish.

2. **Microbiome research:** The study of the microbiome's influence on development and health using Zebrafish provides information on the microbiome's involvement in human disorders.

PRACTICE QUESTIONS

1. Describe the different routes that are used in Zebrafish for drug delivery.
2. What are the advantages and limitations of different routes in drug delivery?
3. Briefly discuss about the procedure of giving *i.p., i.m.,* intrathoracic injection in Zebrafish.
4. What is the angle of various routes used for drug administration in Zebrafish?

REFERENCES

[1]   Hedaya MA. Routes of drug administration. Pharmaceutics. Elsevier 2024; pp. 537-54.
        [http://dx.doi.org/10.1016/B978-0-323-99796-6.00006-0]

[2]   Chaoul V, Dib EY, Bedran J, *et al.* Assessing drug administration techniques in zebrafish models of neurological disease. Int J Mol Sci 2023; 24(19): 14898.
        [http://dx.doi.org/10.3390/ijms241914898] [PMID: 37834345]

[3]   Schroeder PG, Sneddon LU. Exploring the efficacy of immersion analgesics in zebrafish using an integrative approach. Appl Anim Behav Sci 2017; 187: 93-102.
        [http://dx.doi.org/10.1016/j.applanim.2016.12.003]

[4]   Ochocki AJ, Kenney JW. A gelatin-based feed for precise and non-invasive drug delivery to adult zebrafish. J Exp Biol 2023; 226(2): jeb245186.
        [http://dx.doi.org/10.1242/jeb.245186] [PMID: 36606734]

[5]   Stewart A, Cachat JM, Suciu C, *et al.*, Intraperitoneal injection as a method of psychotropic drug delivery in adult zebrafish. Zebrafish neurobehavioral protocols, 2011: p. 169-179.
        [http://dx.doi.org/10.1007/978-1-60761-953-6_14]

[6]   Bise T, Jaźwińska A. Intrathoracic injection for the study of adult zebrafish heart. J Vis Exp, 2019(147).

CHAPTER 3

Blood Collection Methods in Zebrafish

Nileshwar Kalia[1], Ayansh Kaushik[1] and Shamsher Singh[1,*]

[1] Neuropharmacology Division, Department of Pharmacology, ISF College of Pharmacy, Moga, Punjab 142001, India

INTRODUCTION

Aim: To perform the blood collection methods in Zebrafish.

Scope and Outcomes: This chapter covers a thorough examination of Zebrafish blood collection techniques with the goal of clarifying the steps involved and the results that are necessary to progress biomedical research. It will discuss a variety of techniques, including the tail transection method, cardiac puncture, and micro-capillary tube from the dorsal aorta, and will offer thorough guidance on performing these procedures successfully. By following these detailed protocols, researchers will obtain more reproducible results in their Zebrafish studies.

Theory: A crucial area of study in both clinical medicine and biomedical research is hematology, or the study of blood and its problems. *Danio rerio* commonly known as a Zebra fish is endemic to South Asia and crops up as a treasure model for studying the hematological process, due to their genetic tractability and physiological similarities to humans [1, 2]. They are perfect for hematological studies due to their number of benefits. These benefits include that they are transparent in their early stages of growth, which allows the researcher to directly visualize the blood and blood vessels under the microscope without the need for intrusive operations [3]. This transparency makes it easier to image blood cell formation and circulation in real time, providing valuable information about the earliest phases of hematopoiesis. The maximum amount of blood collected in Zebrafish is described in Table **3.1**.

Table 3.1. Blood collection volume in different age groups of Zebrafish.

S. No.	Type of Zebrafish	Maximum Blood Collection Volume
1.	Juvenile Zebrafish	Collect up to 1% of body weight, not exceeding 10μl.
2.	Adult Zebrafish	Collect up to 2% of body weight, not exceeding 100μl.

* Corresponding author Shamsher Singh: Neuropharmacology Division, Department of Pharmacology, ISF College of Pharmacy, Moga, Punjab 142001, India; Tel: +91-9779980588; E-mail: shamshersinghbajwa@gmail.com

Blood collection from the Zebrafish is necessary for research on hematopoiesis, evaluating drug toxicity and efficacy, and genetic and environmental effects on the blood parameters [4, 5]. It contains a blood volume in the range of 8-10% of its total body weight, which is about 0.6-0.7 ml of blood per gram of body weight [6]. A single Zebrafish yields blood volume between 1-10 microliters. There are numerous techniques for collecting the blood from Zebrafish.

These techniques are:

1. Tail transection method
2. Cardiac Puncture
3. Micro capillary tube from dorsal aorta

REQUIREMENTS

Animal: Zebrafish

Chemicals: MS-222, Sterile Water, micro-capillary tube, eugenol.

PROCEDURE

Tail Transection Method

First, all the necessary materials were gathered and the work area was prepared under sterile conditions to avoid any contamination. Zebrafish were carefully selected for the procedure, ensuring that all were in optimal health and condition for sampling.

Anesthetized the Zebrafish using an appropriate anesthetic agent at the recommended concentration. Commonly used anesthetic agents are MS-222 and Eugenol. The depth of anaesthesia needed to immobilize the fish should be sufficient, but not excessive.

Method of Anesthesia

Prepare the stock solution of MS-222 (0.4 grams in one lit.) and dilute it to necessary conditions.

Place the zebrafish in a container filled with the anesthetic solution.

Monitor the fish closely for signs of anesthesia, such as loss of equilibrium, reduced opercula movement, and lack of response to external stimuli, like touch.

Now, transfer the anesthetized fish to a suitable container or petri dish filled with the anesthetic solution. Ensure that the fish is properly oriented and positioned so that the tail fin is easily accessible.

At the distal end of the tail fin, quickly make a transverse incision using sterilized surgical scissors or micro scissors as shown in Fig. (**3.1**).

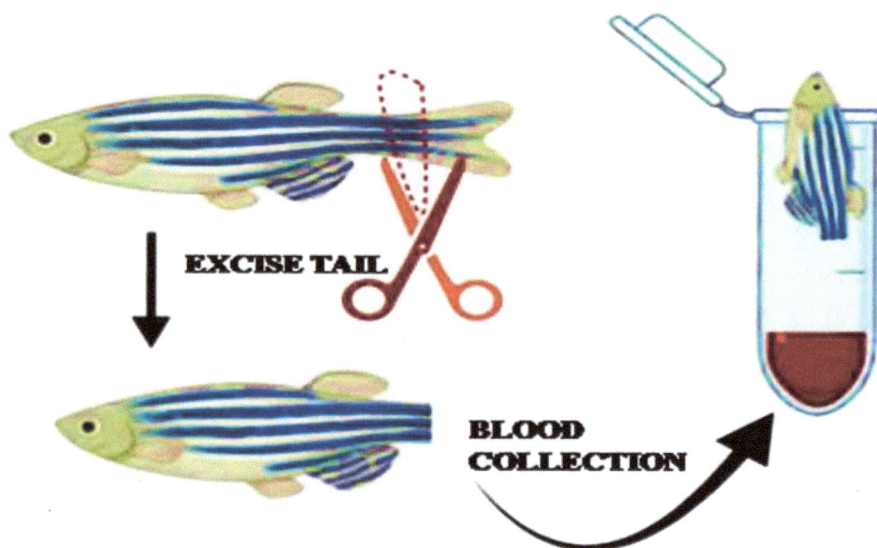

Fig. (3.1). Tail transection method.

To prevent excessive bleeding and stress to the fish, the incision should be made precisely and shallowly. Due to capillary action, blood will naturally pool at the incision time.

To collect the blood, gently position the micro-capillary tube close to the incision site as soon as the cut is made. Allow capillary action to fill the micro-capillary tube with blood. During this process, be careful not to disturb the fish too much.

After collecting enough blood (usually a small amount compared to the size of the fish, taking ethical considerations into account) remove the micro-capillary tube.

Transfer the drawn blood from the micro-capillary tube into a labeled micro-centrifuge tube or another appropriate container with sterile saline solution for analysis or storage.

To stop any bleeding, gently massage the tail fin incision with sterile gauze or a cotton swab. Observe the fish closely for signs of recovery from anesthesia. Move the zebra fish to a freshwater tank that meets the appropriate temperature and water quality standards. Monitor the fish closely for signs of distress or abnormal behavior during the recovery period.

Cardiac Puncture Method

Prepare a solution of 0.16% MS-222 in sterile water.

To anesthetize the Zebrafish, 0.1ml solution of MS-222 per liter of tank water is added to the tank.

Closely monitor the fish to see the signs of anaesthesia, like reduced opercula movement and loss of external stimuli. Once the Zebrafish is anesthetized, carefully transfer it to a paper towel or damp sponge to keep the fish wet under a dissecting microscope.

To expose the ventral surface, gently position the fish so that the ventral side comes up by using sterile forceps.

Just posterior to the operculum, the beating heart is identified. Now insert a micro-capillary tube rinsed with heparin (to prevent blood clotting) *via* the thoracic body cavity into the pericardial cavity. The micro-capillary tube has been directed towards the ventral side of the heart by avoiding the major blood vessels.

The micro-capillary tube is allowed to fill with blood through the capillary action. Do not apply excessive suction of blood, as it causes injury to the heart.

After obtaining enough blood (usually 1–5 µl), gently move the micro-capillary tube to an Eppendorf tube that has been labelled and has 5 µl of sterile phosphate buffer in it.

Now the Eppendorf tube is placed on ice to prevent degradation and coagulation of the sample. Zebrafish should be placed in fresh aerated water, to recover from the anaesthesia (Fig. **3.2**).

Micro-Capillary Tube Method from Dorsal Aorta

Anesthetize the zebra fish and make sure that the fish is fully anesthetized and immobilized.

Now transfer the fish into the dissection dish, containing phosphate buffer solution under the dissection microscope.

To expose the dorsal surface, gently position the fish so that the dorsal side comes up, by using the sterile forceps.

Find the dorsal aorta under the dissecting microscope, it is usually seen as a dark red line that runs along the dorsal midline of the fish.

A micro-capillary tube can be made ready for blood vessel puncturing, by heating and pulling, it to create a fine suitable tip.

Using the micro-capillary tube, carefully puncture the dorsal aorta located just posterior to the anal pore. The angle of insertion should be shallow to avoid damage to other tissues.

Capillary action and arterial pressure help the blood to flow into the micro-capillary tube and collect the desired volume in micro-litres.

Withdraw the micro-capillary tube, after collecting the blood sample.

The Zebrafish should be placed in fresh aerated water, to recover from the anaesthesia (Fig. **3.2**).

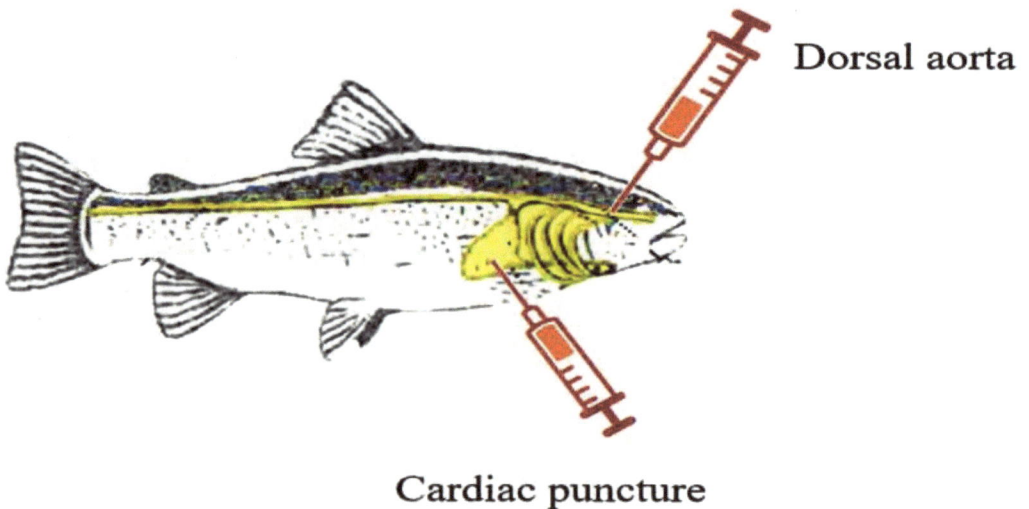

Dorsal aorta

Cardiac puncture

Fig. (3.2). Cardiac puncture and dorsal aorta blood collection method.

APPLICATIONS

1. **Haematological Studies:** Researchers can examine various hematopoietic (the development of blood cells)-related topics in Zebrafish by collecting blood. The blood cells that are investigated include erythrocyte, leukocytes, and thrombocytes as well as their development, differentiation, and maturation [7].
2. **Disease Modelling and Pathophysiology:** Human blood disorders such as anaemia, leukaemia, thrombosis, and immune-related conditions, can be modelled in zebrafish through genetic manipulation [8]. By collecting blood,

scientists can track the progression of these illnesses by identifying the biomarkers and underlying molecular pathways.

3. **Genetic and Molecular Studies:** Blood samples include genetic material (DNA and RNA) that can be examined to learn more about the regulatory systems, gene expression patterns, and mutations that affect the growth and function of blood cells [9]. This is helpful in finding the therapeutic targets for haematological disorders.

4. **Regenerative Medicines:** Zebrafish are capable of regeneration [10]. This includes tissue and blood cell regeneration. It helps the researchers to investigate the mechanism of hematopoietic regeneration.

5. **Drug Discovery and Toxicology:** Blood samples from zebrafish are crucial for evaluating the efficacy and toxicity of pharmaceutical compounds [4]. Researchers can assess how drugs affect haematological parameters, such as haematocrit, haemoglobin levels, and immune cell function.

LIMITATIONS

1. Zebrafish are small animals, and their total volume is limited. This restricts the volume of blood that can be extracted from a single fish without causing stress to their health. Ethical criteria governing the maximum blood volume permitted in relation to fish size must be followed by researchers.

2. Blood collection from zebrafish requires precise skills and techniques.

3. Zebrafish have a very short life span (2-3 years), which may restrict the feasibility of long-term studies.

4. Environmental factors like temperature changes, chemical exposure, and water quality have an impact on Zebrafish. If these variables are not properly controlled, they may affect the haematological parameters.

PRACTICE QUESTIONS

1. Why is blood collected from the Zebrafish in research?
2. What are common methods used to collect blood from Zebrafish?
3. Why is anaesthesia important during blood collection from Zebrafish?
4. What are some challenges associated with Zebrafish blood collection?
5. What are the ethical considerations when collecting blood from Zebrafish?

REFERENCES

[1]   Whiteley AR, Bhat A, Martins EP, *et al.* Population genomics of wild and laboratory zebrafish (*Danio rerio*). Mol Ecol 2011; 20(20): 4259-76.
      [http://dx.doi.org/10.1111/j.1365-294X.2011.05272.x] [PMID: 21923777]

[2]   Howe K, Clark MD, Torroja CF, *et al.* The zebrafish reference genome sequence and its relationship to the human genome. Nature 2013; 496(7446): 498-503.
      [http://dx.doi.org/10.1038/nature12111] [PMID: 23594743]

[3]   Zhao S, Huang J, Ye J. A fresh look at zebrafish from the perspective of cancer research. J Exp Clin Cancer Res 2015; 34(1): 80.
[http://dx.doi.org/10.1186/s13046-015-0196-8] [PMID: 26260237]

[4]   Kari G, Rodeck U, Dicker AP. Zebrafish: an emerging model system for human disease and drug discovery. Clin Pharmacol Ther 2007; 82(1): 70-80.
[http://dx.doi.org/10.1038/sj.clpt.6100223] [PMID: 17495877]

[5]   Witeska M, Kondera E, Bojarski B. Hematological and hematopoietic analysis in fish toxicology—a review. Animals (Basel) 2023; 13(16): 2625.
[http://dx.doi.org/10.3390/ani13162625] [PMID: 37627416]

[6]   Zang L, Shimada Y, Nishimura Y, Tanaka T, Nishimura N. Repeated blood collection for blood tests in adult zebrafish 2015.

[7]   de Jong JLO, Zon LI. Use of the zebrafish system to study primitive and definitive hematopoiesis. Annu Rev Genet 2005; 39(1): 481-501.
[http://dx.doi.org/10.1146/annurev.genet.39.073003.095931] [PMID: 16285869]

[8]   Mastrogiovanni M, Martínez-Navarro FJ, Bowman TV, Cayuela ML. Inflammation in development and aging: Insights from the zebrafish model. Int J Mol Sci 2024; 25(4): 2145.
[http://dx.doi.org/10.3390/ijms25042145] [PMID: 38396822]

[9]   Haffter P, Granato M, Brand M, *et al.* The identification of genes with unique and essential functions in the development of the zebrafish, *Danio rerio*. Development 1996; 123(1): 1-36.
[http://dx.doi.org/10.1242/dev.123.1.1] [PMID: 9007226]

[10]   Poss KD, Keating MT, Nechiporuk A. Tales of regeneration in zebrafish. Dev Dyn 2003; 226(2): 202-10.
[http://dx.doi.org/10.1002/dvdy.10220] [PMID: 12557199]

CHAPTER 4

Anesthesia Techniques in Zebrafish

Kousik Maparu[1], Falguni Goel[1] and Shamsher Singh[1,*]

[1] *Neuropharmacology Division, Department of Pharmacology, ISF College of Pharmacy, Moga, Punjab 142001, India*

INTRODUCTION

Aim: To study anesthesia techniques in adult Zebrafish.

Scope and outcomes: Anesthesia is necessary for various scientific and veterinary treatments involving Zebrafish(*Danio rerio*). Effective anesthetic techniques guarantee minimal stress and discomfort to the fish while enabling experimental manipulations, surgeries, and other treatments.

Theory: Anesthesia is commonly used in fish experiments, but using an insufficient anesthetic technique may harm the reliability of the data as well as the well-being of the animals. In recent years, Zebrafish (*Danio rerio*) have been used more frequently in biomedical research, emphasizing the significance of using appropriate anesthetic regimens for these species. Although the primary anesthetic medications along with a few analgesic techniques have been identified, further study is required before they can be applied to this species. A systematized observation of indicators is also recommended to assess the welfare of adult Zebrafish and minimize their pain [1].

General anesthesia in fish can be induced by diluting anesthetics in water, where they are absorbed primarily through the intestines. However, in some species, it can be absorbed through the skin [2]. Factors such as the method of administration, salinity, pH, temperature, nitrogenous substances, oxygenation, and other environmental parameters can influence how anesthesia affects fish [3]. Additionally, variables including length of anesthesia, concentration of anesthetics, body weight, metabolism of the fish, gill surface, health of the fish, age, strain, and the unique characteristics of each species of fish all affect the depth and recovery of anesthesia. As a result, before protocols are established, anesthesia trials with a limited number of fish or pilot studies must be carried out to ascertain the ideal dosage and exposure duration.

* **Corresponding author Shamsher Singh:** Neuropharmacology Division, Department of Pharmacology, ISF College of Pharmacy, Moga, Punjab 142001, India; Tel: +91-9779980588; E-mail: shamshersinghbajwa@gmail.com

Stages of Anesthesia in Zebrafish

A total of 8 phases were observed in Zebrafish after giving anesthesia [4] (Fig. **4.1**).

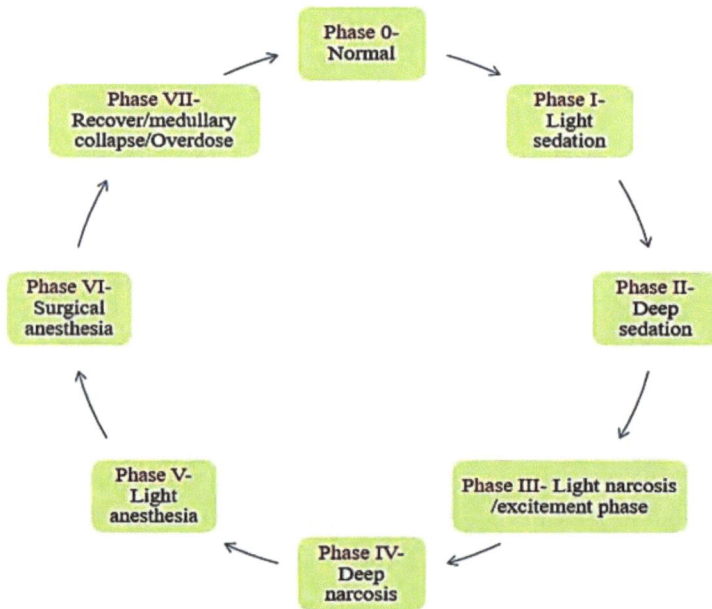

Fig. (4.1). Stages of anesthesia in Zebrafish.

1. **Phase 0-Normal:** Normal muscle tone, normal respiratory rate, and normal reaction to visual and tactile stimuli.
2. **Phase I-Light sedation:** Little reduction in response to touch and visual cues.
3. **Phase II-Deep sedation:** There is a minor decrease in respiration rate and muscle tone, with no response to light touch or visual stimulation.
4. **Phase III- Light Narcosis/Excitement Phase:** This phase is characterized by a partial loss of stability, poor reactions to postural changes, decreased muscle tone, and heightened sensitivity to touch and visual stimuli. Furthermore, there is either erratic breathing or an increase in the respiratory rate.
5. **Phase IV-Deep Narcosis:** Complete loss of equilibrium is present, along with no reactivity to small touch or visual cues or to changes in posture. The rate of breathing was close to normal.
6. **Phase V-Light Anesthesia:** Complete loss of muscular tone is present, along with a drop in heart and breathing rates and no response to unpleasant stimuli.
7. **Phase VI-Surgical Anesthesia:** Extremely low respiratory and slow cardiac rates are present, along with no response to intense stimulus.
8. **Phase VII-Recover/Medullary Collapse/Overdose:** After some time, fish will

recover or apnea is accompanied by a limping, non-respiratory tone that can cause cardiac arrest in a matter of minutes if the level of anesthesia is not rapidly reduced. In the end, this illness may be fatal.

Commonly Used Anesthetic Agents

Table 4.1. Commonly used anesthetic agents used for anesthesia in Zebrafish [4, 5].

S. No.	Anesthetic agents	Concentration	Preparation	Dosage for Different Phases	Induction Time	Recovery	Usage	Advantages	Disadvantages
01	Tricaine methanesuifonate (MS-222)	Typically used at 100-200 mg/L for anesthesia and 300-500 mg/L for euthanasia.	MS-222 is acidic and should be buffered to a neutral pH (7.0-7.5) using sodium bicarbonate.	**Stage V** - 100, 120, 140, 160, 180 and 200 mg/L (Immersion) **Stage III-IV** -100 and 120 mg/L (Immersion) **Stage V** - 140, 160, 180 and 200 mg/L (Immersion) **Stage VI** 150 mg/L (Immersion)	Anesthesia is usually achieved within 2-3 minutes	Fish typically recover within 5-10 minutes when placed in fresh water.	The most commonly used anesthetic for Zebrafish	Effective, readily available, and well-documented.	Requires careful pH adjustment and monitoring.
02	Eugenol (Clove Oil)	Typically used at 20-100 mg/L	Must be mixed with ethanol to dissolve in water for inhalation.	**Stage V** - 60, 80, 100, 120 and 140 mg/L (Immersion)	Anesthesia is generally achieved within 2-3 minutes	Fish recover within 5-10 minutes in fresh water.	An economical and effective alternative for Zebrafish anesthesia	Inexpensive and readily available.	Potential for variability in concentration and effectiveness; can be irritating at high concentrations.
03	Isoflurane	Typically used at 3-5% solution.	Fish are exposed to a saturated solution of Isoflurane in water or bubbled into the water.	**Stage I** 300 mg/L (Immersion) **Stage VI** 325 mg/L (Immersion) **Stage VI/VII** 350 mg/L (Immersion)	Rapid, usually within a minute.	Quick recovery upon transfer to fresh water.	An alternative to MS-222, used primarily for short procedures.	Non-irritating and easy to administer.	Limited solubility in water, requiring specialized equipment for administration.
04	Metomi-date hydrochloride	Typically, 2 - 4 mg/L is used.	Used as inhalant anaesth-etic in a water bath in fish.	**Stage I** 2 and 4 mg/L (Immersion) **Stage IV** 6, 8 and 10 mg/L (Immersion)	Light anesthesia occurs between 2.3 and 4.3 min.	Recover in 2.8 min to 5.2 min.	Used for minor procedures.	No distressful behaviour observed during anesthesia. No mortality was seen during or after anesthesia.	Does not induce a surgical anaesthetic stage or analgesia, alter fish physiology by suppressing cortisol production.

(Table 4.1) cont.....

S. No.	Anesthetic agents	Concentration	Preparation	Dosage for Different Phases	Induction Time	Recovery	Usage	Advantages	Disadvantages
05	Ketamine	Typically used at 2000mg/L	Can be injected or used in an anesthetic bath	**Stage IV** (at least) 8000 mg/L (Immersion)	Induces anesthesia quickly, especially when combined with medetomidine.	Longer recovery time (up to 24 minutes) when used with medetomidine.	Effective for inducing surgical anesthesia.	Decreased gill movement, and decreased stress response to hypoxia and repeated administration of ketamine do not cause tolerance or sensitization to specific drug effects.	Ketamine revealed to be neurotoxic to Zebrafish larvae.

REQUIREMENTS

Animal: Adult Zebrafish

Equipment: Petri dish, Anesthetics, ice bath, *etc.*

GENERAL PROCEDURE FOR ANESTHESIA

1. Fill an empty anesthetic tank with one liter of system water.
2. Add 150 mg of MS-222 and 300 mg of baking soda (in a ratio of 1:2) and mix properly. And verify that the solution's pH falls between 6-7.
3. Fill a second empty tank (the recovery tank) with 1 liter of system water.
4. Take the Zebrafish out of the home tank and put them straight into the anesthesia tank using a dry, disinfected fish-holding net.
5. Monitor the fish for signs of opercula movement and lack of the ability to correct itself usually occurs within 1-2 minutes.
6. Pinch the tail fin. A surgical plane of anesthesia is reached when the tail fin pinch elicits no reaction response.
7. Return fish to their recovery tank and wait for the recovery of behavior and physiological functions.

ANESTHETIC TECHNIQUES

Immersion Anesthesia

Immersion anesthesia is a [7] method of providing anesthesia in which the patient or fish is completely immersed in a liquid anesthetic substance rather than inhaling it or getting it intravenously. This method was mostly employed in the early days of anesthesia exploration, particularly prior to the creation of safer and more regulated administration techniques, such as intravenous and inhalation anesthesia.

Method: The most common technique involves immersing Zebrafish in a solution containing an anesthetic agent.

Procedure: Prepare an anesthetic solution at the appropriate concentration.

The fish were placed in the solution and monitored until they reached the desired level of anesthesia.

For recovery, the fish were transferred to fresh water and monitored until they regained their normal behavior.

Inhalation Anesthesia

During experimental treatments, inhalation anesthesia [8] in Zebrafish refers to the induction and maintenance of anesthesia in these aquatic creatures using volatile anesthetics such as isoflurane.

Method: Less commonly used, involving the administration of gaseous anesthetics such as isoflurane.

Procedure: Saturate the water with the gaseous anesthetic or bubble it into the water.

Place the fish in anesthetic-infused water.

The concentration was monitored and adjusted as needed.

Anesthesia by Cooling

Fish's movements and overall metabolic activity, including their excretion of ammonia and feces, are slowed down when water is gradually cooled. In addition to lowering oxygen consumption, this metabolic rate reduction increases the ability of water to retain dissolved oxygen.

However, unlike the total blockage observed with MS-222, nerve conduction was only somewhat reduced, depending on the species. Therefore, it is not advisable to use a cooling anesthetic during invasive procedures. Although it works well to immobilize fish, it is usually regarded as insufficient on its own as an anesthetic. Rapid cooling, on the other hand, causes fatal shock and probably interferes with osmoregulatory processes. Anesthesia of fish using cold water is depicted in Fig. (**4.2**) [9].

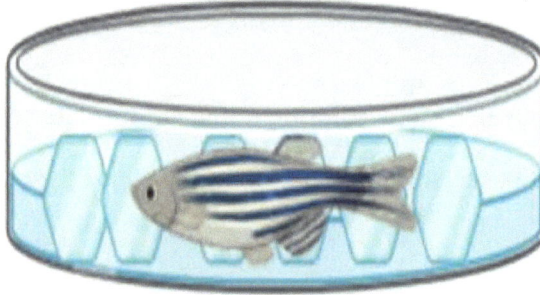

Fig. (4.2). Anesthesia of Zebrafish using ice water.

MONITORING AND SAFETY

1. **Depth of anesthesia**: Assessed by observing the fish's response to stimuli (*e.g.*, fin movement and gill movement).
2. **Water quality**: Ensure that water quality parameters (temperature, pH, and oxygen levels) are within appropriate ranges to minimize stress.
3. **Recovery**: Place the fish in clean, well-oxygenated water for recovery. Monitor until normal swimming and behavior are restored.
4. **Handling**: Minimize handling time and avoid rough manipulation to reduce stress and potential injuries.

CONSIDERATIONS

1. **Species-Specific Responses**: Anesthetic sensitivity can vary among different strains and developmental stages of Zebrafish.
2. **Experimental Requirements**: Choose the anesthetic agent and method based on the specific requirements of the procedure and the required duration of anesthesia.
3. **Ethical Practices**: Ensure that all procedures are conducted following ethical guidelines and institutional animal care protocols.

By carefully selecting and administering anesthetics, researchers can ensure the humane treatment of Zebrafish while achieving effective immobilization for various scientific and veterinary purposes.

PRACTICE QUESTIONS

1. What is anesthesia?
2. What anesthetics are used for Zebrafish?
3. What are the anesthesia procedures for Zebrafish?
4. What is the safety monitoring taken during the anesthesia procedure?
5. What is the general procedure for anesthesia in Zebrafish?

REFERENCES

[1]   Collymore C, Tolwani A, Lieggi C, Rasmussen S. Efficacy and safety of 5 anesthetics in adult zebrafish (*Danio rerio*). J Am Assoc Lab Anim Sci 2014; 53(2): 198-203.
[PMID: 24602548]

[2]   Chatigny F, Kamunde C, Creighton CM, Stevens ED. Uses and doses of local anesthetics in fish, amphibians, and reptiles. J Am Assoc Lab Anim Sci 2017; 56(3): 244-53.
[PMID: 28535859]

[3]   Neiffer DL, Stamper MA. Fish sedation, analgesia, anesthesia, and euthanasia: considerations, methods, and types of drugs. ILAR J 2009; 50(4): 343-60.
[http://dx.doi.org/10.1093/ilar.50.4.343] [PMID: 19949251]

[4]   Martins T, Valentim AM, Pereira N, Antunes LM. Anaesthesia and analgesia in laboratory adult zebrafish: A question of refinement. Lab Anim 2016; 50(6): 476-88.
[http://dx.doi.org/10.1177/0023677216670686] [PMID: 27909198]

[5]   von Krogh K, Higgins J, Saavedra Torres Y, Mocho JP. Screening of anaesthetics in adult zebrafish (*Danio rerio*) for the induction of euthanasia by overdose. Biology (Basel) 2021; 10(11): 1133.
[http://dx.doi.org/10.3390/biology10111133] [PMID: 34827125]

[6]   Owen JP, Kelsh RN. A suitable anaesthetic protocol for metamorphic zebrafish. PLoS One 2021; 16(3): e0246504.
[http://dx.doi.org/10.1371/journal.pone.0246504] [PMID: 33667238]

[7]   Schroeder PG, Sneddon LU. Exploring the efficacy of immersion analgesics in zebrafish using an integrative approach. Appl Anim Behav Sci 2017; 187: 93-102.
[http://dx.doi.org/10.1016/j.applanim.2016.12.003]

[8]   Ferreira JT, Schoonbee HJ, Smit GL. The uptake of the anaesthetic benzocaine hydrochloride by the gills and the skin of three freshwater fish species. J Fish Biol 1984; 25(1): 35-41.
[http://dx.doi.org/10.1111/j.1095-8649.1984.tb04848.x]

[9]   Chen K, Wang CQ, Fan YQ, *et al.* The evaluation of rapid cooling as an anesthetic method for the zebrafish. Zebrafish 2014; 11(1): 71-5.
[http://dx.doi.org/10.1089/zeb.2012.0858] [PMID: 24093489]

CHAPTER 5

Shoaling Behaviour in Zebrafish

Pratyush Porel[1] and **Shamsher Singh**[1,*]

[1] *Neuropharmacology Division, Department of Pharmacology, ISF College of Pharmacy, Moga, Punjab 142001, India*

INTRODUCTION

Aim: To study the shoaling behaviour in adult Zebrafish.

Scope and outcomes: Shoaling behaviour is a social interaction behavior where animals make social perceptions with other individuals followed by forming a group or schools to move together. A shoaling behaviour test is performed to evaluate the neurobehavioral parameters of Zebrafish.

Theory; Zebrafish as a Model to Study Behavioral Neuroscience:

Zebrafish is a tropical teleost, small fish, mainly found in freshwater. After 1970, Zebrafish became a widely accepted novel animal model for biomedical research purposes, including behavioral, genetic and ecotoxicological studies. The brain of Zebrafish shows a greater extent of similarities with the human brain in psychopharmacological and neurobehavioral aspects, so different neurological diseases can be studied by inducing that particular disease in Zebrafish. Over the commonly used animal models, including rodents, drosophila and *C. elegans*, Zebrafish makes itself feasible from some natural perspectives like its small size, availability, maintenance, acquisition and ease of taking care. Additionally, Zebrafish are highly similar in anatomical, and physiological prospects to mammals, which gives them more preference to establish themselves as animal model for biomedical research [1]. The average life span of Zebrafish is around 4-5 years whereas at the age of 10-12 weeks, the fish become reproductively mature and capable of laying 200-300 eggs per week. Generally, female fish are capable of reproducing every 2-3 days, and each clutch laid by them may contain several hundred eggs which give birth to hundreds of caviars. Within 3 months, fish become mature enough to be used in various experiments as an animal model [2]. Nowadays, Zebrafish are a prime model for studying genetics, mutagenetic

---

* **Corresponding author Shamsher Singh:** Neuropharmacology Division, Department of Pharmacology, ISF College of Pharmacy, Moga, Punjab 142001, India; Tel: +91-9779980588; E-mail: shamshersinghbajwa@gmail.com

screening and toxicology. In recent decades, an exact explanation of the pathophysiology of multifaceted behavioural disorders has been a main goal for researchers and Zebrafish provides an immense opportunity to study the basic functions of the brain through behavioural studies. Undoubtedly, rodents possess a closer anatomical structure to the human brain, but their complexity and expensive maintenance, provide more advantages to Zebrafish in establishing themself successfully as an alternative animal model. Zebrafish is also very much feasible for high throughput screening (HTS) methods for drug development in neuroscience, whereas rodent models may not be suitable for the same due to high maintenance [3].

According to taxonomical classifications, there are uncountable species around the world that express more intraspecies interaction. This is called preference for conspecifics. Previously, there were some attempts to use shoaling behaviour as a behavioural measure, but no standardized protocol or model has been established to study this. Adult Zebrafish and larvae are now widely used in the study of neurobehavioral parameters and shoaling nature. In simple words, "shoal" means, a group or aggregation of individuals and "school" means, shoals exhibiting polarized and synchronized motion. Shoaling behaviour is complex and dynamic behaviour, which is a characteristic behaviour that is predominantly observed in Zebrafish. Some behaviors are characterized by aggression, fear, alarm reaction, sleep and reward by studying the shoaling behaviour of Zebrafish. Due to some advantages like ease of breeding, handling and practical simplicity, its application is increasing as a translational tool in the drug discovery process [4].

REQUIREMENTS

Animal: Adult Zebrafish

Apparatus: Normal glass tank, Any-maze software, Graph-pad-prism, Camera

SHOALING BEHAVIOUR IN ZEBRAFISH

Behaviour is a complex phenomenon that possesses a core relationship with neurobiological mechanisms. Interaction with others and the expression of social perception are essential for all species to survive in the animal kingdom. Social behaviour can be expressed as foraging, aggression, competition and mating. Currently, several researches are ongoing to check animal behaviour and their mechanisms, and studies are designed in such a manner that correlate the nature of animal behaviour with human beings. Zebrafish spend most of their life in small, firm gatherings, called shoals and exhibit shoaling behaviour by synchronizing swimming in one direction, which is illustrated in Fig. (**5.1**). Zebrafish's shoaling nature develops slowly from about 7 days to adulthood.

Depending on the situation, circumstances and physiological conditions, shoal may tighten or loosen. Anxiety or fear causes the shoal to tighten and potentially form a school. Shoal becomes looser and its organization becomes less oriented if stimulation comes in the form of hunger or habituation. This behaviour can be observed manually and using automated video-recording software. The focal coordinates, which are used for tracking fish's movements by video recording software are diagrammatically represented in Fig. (**5.2**). Several endpoints are accessed as a goal of study including the inter-fish distance shown in Fig. (**5.3**), shoal area, nearest and farthest neighbor distances shown in Fig. (**5.4**), total time spent in the shoal and away from the shoal, and the number of animals leaving the shoal and polarization. Some neurological diseases like anxiety, depression, epilepsy and traumatic brain injury (TBI) significantly affect the shoaling behaviour of Zebrafish [5].

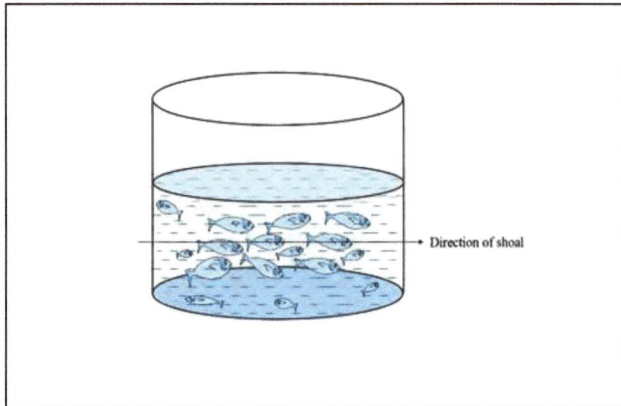

Fig. (5.1). Shoaling behavior and its direction.

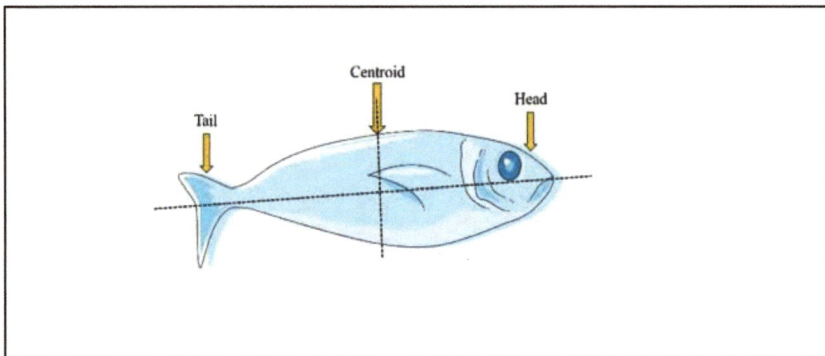

Fig. (5.2). Coordinates (head, centroid and tail) for the focal fish tracking system.

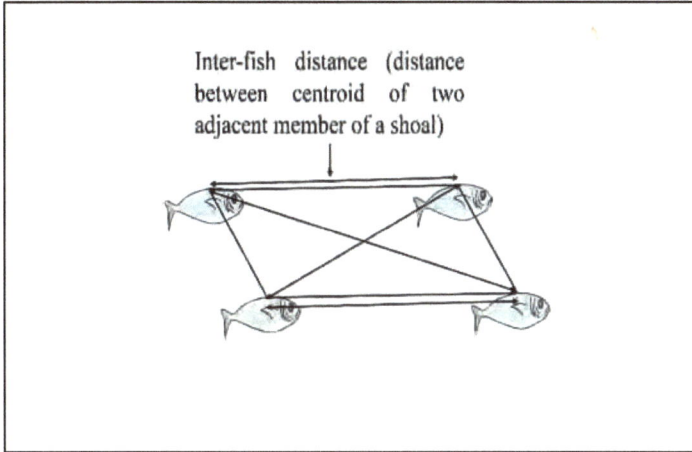

Fig. (5.3). Measurement of inter-fish distance.

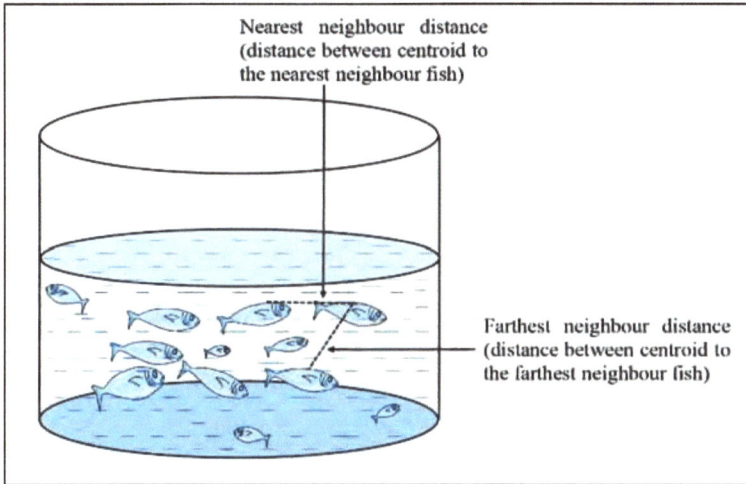

Fig. (5.4). Measurement of nearest and farthest neighborhood distance.

Factors Affecting the Shoaling Behavior in Zebrafish

There are several factors that are enlisted for affecting the shoaling behaviour of Zebrafish. Overall, factors can be categorized into two major groups such as biotic factors and abiotic factors. In the following sections, some factors are discussed that impart smaller to larger effects on the shoaling behaviour of Zebrafish.

Temperature of Water

Temperature is the most important and major abiotic factor of all. There are so many studies being performed to check the effects of temperature on behaviour of fish. The effects of temperature on the growth, metabolism and reproduction of fish are well reported but limitation arises in the study of neuropharmacology. An increase in surrounding temperature as well as water temperature decreases anxiety and increases the time spent in the brighter area and danger zone. The shoals of Zebrafish also become loose as the temperature increases, and fish are likely to be present in smaller groups. Thermal tolerance and the impact of temperature on the central nervous system (CNS) are not well defined, so further research is required in this field [6].

pH of Water

The pH of water is another important abiotic factor that needs to be discussed after temperature. In most of the average-grade laboratory and Zebrafish husbandry, normal running water is used to keep them in tanks. This water does not belong to the optimum pH range and may be checked rarely. A study reveals that small changes in pH are enough to cause an alteration in the locomotor activity of fish. Very few studies are reported about the effect of pH on shoaling behaviour, that is why it could be an open field of research for researchers [7].

Tank Size

Tank size is also an abiotic factor. In the middle of a water tank, transparent and opaque plates are placed close to each other. The depth of the water is measured (7-8 cm). The fish which is under experiment is not well acquainted with how to form the shoal. This fish is placed in front of the opaque plate and another 10 fish are placed in front of the transparent plate. The only way to pass from one chamber to another is through the funnel but initially, the fish is prevented from entering another side. The test fish is placed inside the tank for 2 minutes to adapt to the environment and then the opaque plate is removed. The total time is noted from removing the opaque plate to joining the shoal after passing through the funnel to the other side. So, in larger areas, Zebrafish make shoals more readily than in smaller areas [8].

Flow of Water

Zebrafish show shoaling behaviour by swimming in a synchronized way in a particular direction. The ability to swim directly or indirectly hinges on the direction of flow and flow rate. Shoaling behaviour depends upon the water flow because Zebrafish tend to form smaller shoals in still water as compared to fast-moving water [9].

Influence of Sex and Phenotype

Preference for similar sex and phenotype are considered biotic factors. Another advantage of forming shoals is to protect themselves from the attack of predators. Due to this reason, Zebrafish form shoals with similar sex and phenotypic individuals. So that the predator will face difficulty in identifying the specific target fish. The shoaling behaviour also provides the benefit from predators to both males and females, and it is always noted both sexes do not make the same decisions regarding the shoaling, including the shoal size, inter shoal distances, shoal area *etc.* In a study, males and females of each type of *Danio rerio* (wild type, golden mutants and leopard mutants) and another species of pearl danios are taken, and studies were performed to check their shoaling behaviour and whether they are making shoals with the individual of their own species or with the dissimilar species. According to the hypothesis of prioritizing the identical sexes and similar species, the fish typically identified their shoal mates with the same sexes and conspecifics. This result validates the impact of prioritizing similar sex and phenotypes in the shoaling behaviour of Zebrafish [10].

Research Outcomes on Shoaling Behaviour

Alcohol

An addictive substance, like alcohol, imparts a very serious effect on an animal's behaviour. The sedative properties of alcohol are also attributed to its effect on the neurochemical system (GABAergic system, dopamine and serotonin levels) in adult animals. Some recent studies have already been performed with the aim of screening the effect of alcohol on shoaling behaviour. Acute administration of ethyl alcohol exerts a significant effect on shoaling behaviour. Alcohol-disordered polarization of animals significantly reduced their shoal behaviour. Alcohol exposure during fatal development causes a teratogenic effect and significantly alters foetus development. As many studies have reported that the effect of ethanol on Zebrafish is dose-dependent, lower to moderate doses (0-0.5%) of ethanol increase locomotor activity and shoaling behaviour, including nearest shoal distance and shoal area whereas, higher doses (1.0%) of ethanol decrease locomotor activity, shoal distance and shoal area. Acute or chronic administration of ethanol (0.5%) significantly increases the inter-fish distance and area. Overall, treatment with alcohol at a lower to moderate dose exerts anxiolytic behaviour and that's why increased social interaction or shoaling [11].

Caffeine

Caffeine is a centrally acting drug that evokes stimulatory responses in rodents and Zebrafish. Dose-dependent responses to caffeine are also reported in both mammals and Zebrafish. A high dose of caffeine shows an anxiety-like state with no alteration in locomotor behaviours. Studies have indicated that caffeine administration at higher doses (25, 50 mg/L) increases shoaling behaviour compared to the lower dose (5 mg/L). A much higher dose (100 mg/L) exposure for 15 minutes decreased shoal volume, shoal area and inter-shoal distance. Thus, it concludes that caffeine increases anxiety and shoaling in Zebrafish [12].

Quercetin

Quercetin is a flavonoid that is found in various green vegetables, fruits and grains. It is also present in food supplements of fish. The conventional uses of quercetin as an antioxidant, anti-inflammatory and anticancer agent are already established and due to these properties, it is used as a potential additive in fish feed. On the other side, quercetin is reported to cause mutations and DNA strand breaks in some *in vitro* studies. So many studies have also revealed some adverse effects of quercetin. For example, sub-acute intraperitoneal administration of quercetin (50 mg/kg animal body weight) reduced the uptake of radio-labelled iodine and thus thyroid function was interrupted. At low concentrations (between 0.1-60 µM), quercetin promotes estrogenic-mediated carcinogenesis. After metabolism, quercetin is converted into o-semi-quinone and o-quinone, which are reactive oxidative species and can cause cytotoxic effects. As an adverse effect, quercetin causes disruption of blood vessel development in adult Zebrafish and mitochondrial dysfunction, along with impaired locomotor movement in larval *Danio rerio*. These reports are suggested to emphasize more research on the various effects of quercetin on *in vitro* or animal models, including rodents, non-rodents and Zebrafish. In recent decades, some studies have been performed to check the effect of quercetin on the shoaling behaviour of Zebrafish. Based on previous studies, the detrimental effect of quercetin is dose-dependent. At lower concentrations, quercetin has beneficial effects, but the effects are altered with a gradual dose increment. In a study, six graded doses of quercetin were taken and showed beneficial effects on shoaling and anxiety behaviours. At a lower concentration, quercetin increased the shoaling tendency and decreased anxiety. On a higher dose, it shows detrimental effects by decreasing movements and increasing anxiety [13].

APPLICATIONS OF SHOALING BEHAVIOUR AND DISEASE CONDITIONS

1. **Anxiety:** Anxiety is a feeling of worry or any uncertain outcomes. Anxiety may arise due to various reasons both psychological and physiological. Stressful life events, fear of uncertain things, thoughts and trauma are responsible for the development of anxiety in animals. If the animal is suffering

from anxiety, then it will try to make a group or join the group, called shoals, which further reduces its anxiety. Hence, the study of shoaling behaviour also helps to quantify the conditions and behavioural changes in higher animals.

2. **Depression:** Depression is the most common psychiatric condition that is seen in animals as well as humans. In depression, Zebrafish prefer to stay at the corners of the tank rather than form shoals. That indicates depressed conditions, when fish prefer to stay alone as opposed to gathering with others. This type of behavioural change is also noted in humans.

3. **Epilepsy:** Epilepsy is a neuro-electrophysiological disease, commonly characterized by recurrent tremors and seizures. Pentylenetetrazole (PTZ) is commonly used to induce seizures in animals. It is observed that PTZ decreased shoaling behaviour by increasing the inter-fish distance and shoal area and significantly decreasing the shoal cohesion.

4. **Traumatic brain injury:** TBI is one of the major causes of death in developing countries around the world. In the laboratory, artificial mechanical injury is performed in the brains of Zebrafish to mimic the condition of TBI and then shoaling behaviour is observed. In times of trauma, fish show more interest in joining the shoal.

ADVANTAGES

1. The study of shoaling behaviour using Zebrafish, emerging as a novel and widely accepted animal model to study neuropharmacology because it has greater similarities with the human brain.

2. Shoaling behaviour represents the preference for similar sex and phenotypes to make shoals.

3. Shoaling behaviour can be changed in stressful conditions and many diseased conditions as well. So, changes in shoaling behaviour are also a stress indicator.

4. Shoaling behaviour shows a greater relationship with different neuronal diseases such as anxiety, depression, epilepsy and TBI. That's why, it becomes a parameter to be checked during the study of various neurodegenerative diseases.

LIMITATIONS

1. More emphasis should be given to the evaluation of various neurotransmitter levels and synaptic functions in the brain and compared with the clinical events.

2. The effect of temperature, pH and salinity of water on the shoaling behaviour of Zebrafish is not well established. These all should be considered crucial factors to be studied by the researchers.

3. A study should be designed on escape tendency and isolation from shoals on a laboratory scale and correlate with clinical parameters.

4. Statistical analysis of the obtained data for all groups should be performed carefully and a more precise assay method needs to be designed to check the shoaling behaviour.

PRACTICE QUESTIONS

1. Discuss shoaling behaviour briefly.
2. What is the preference for conspecifics?
3. Discuss the effect of sex and phenotype on shoaling behaviour.
4. What are the different disease conditions that modulate shoaling behaviour? Discuss any one of them.
5. Discuss the average nearest neighbour distance and farthest neighbour distance with suitable diagrams.
6. Caffeine increases shoaling behaviour. Will nicotine do the same? Establish your opinion with valid statements.

REFERENCES

[1]   Choi TY, Choi TI, Lee YR, Choe SK, Kim CH. Zebrafish as an animal model for biomedical research. Exp Mol Med 2021; 53(3): 310-7.
        [http://dx.doi.org/10.1038/s12276-021-00571-5] [PMID: 33649498]

[2]   Spence R. Zebrafish ecology and behaviour. Zebrafish models in neurobehavioral research. 2011: 1-46.
        [http://dx.doi.org/10.1007/978-1-60761-922-2_1]

[3]   Patton EE, Zon LI, Langenau DM. Zebrafish disease models in drug discovery: From preclinical modelling to clinical trials. Nat Rev Drug Discov 2021; 20(8): 611-28.
        [http://dx.doi.org/10.1038/s41573-021-00210-8] [PMID: 34117457]

[4]   Buske C. Zebrafish shoaling behavior: Its development, quantification, neuro-chemical correlates, and application in a disease model. Canada: University of Toronto 2013.

[5]   Pagnussat N, Piato AL, Schaefer IC, *et al.* One for all and all for one: The importance of shoaling on behavioral and stress responses in zebrafish. Zebrafish 2013; 10(3): 338-42.
        [http://dx.doi.org/10.1089/zeb.2013.0867] [PMID: 23802189]

[6]   Abozaid A, Tsang B, Gerlai R. The effects of small but abrupt change in temperature on the behavior of larval zebrafish. Physiol Behav 2020; 227: 113169.
        [http://dx.doi.org/10.1016/j.physbeh.2020.113169] [PMID: 32918940]

[7]   Cleal M, Gibbon A, Fontana BD, Parker MO. The importance of pH: How aquarium water is affecting behavioural responses to drug exposure in larval zebrafish. Pharmacol Biochem Behav 2020; 199: 173066.
        [http://dx.doi.org/10.1016/j.pbb.2020.173066] [PMID: 33137371]

[8]   Maierdiyali A, Wang L, Luo Y, Li Z. Effect of tank size on zebrafish behavior and physiology. Animals (Basel) 2020; 10(12): 2353.
        [http://dx.doi.org/10.3390/ani10122353] [PMID: 33317187]

[9]   Miller N, Gerlai R. Quantification of shoaling behaviour in zebrafish (*Danio rerio*). Behav Brain Res 2007; 184(2): 157-66.
        [http://dx.doi.org/10.1016/j.bbr.2007.07.007] [PMID: 17707522]

[10]   Snekser JL, Ruhl N, Bauer K, McRobert SP. The influence of sex and phenotype on shoaling decisions in zebrafish. Int J Comp Psychol 2010; 23(1)

[http://dx.doi.org/10.46867/IJCP.2010.23.01.04]

[11] Araujo-Silva H, Leite-Ferreira ME, Luchiari AC. Behavioral screening of alcohol effects and individual differences in zebrafish (*Danio rerio*). Alcohol Alcohol 2020; 55(6): 591-7.
[http://dx.doi.org/10.1093/alcalc/agaa046] [PMID: 32533153]

[12] Connaughton VP, Clayman CL. Neurochemical and behavioral consequences of ethanol and/or caffeine exposure: Effects in zebrafish and rodents. Curr Neuropharmacol 2022; 20(3): 560-78.
[http://dx.doi.org/10.2174/1570159X19666211111142027] [PMID: 34766897]

[13] Zhang J, Liu M, Cui W, Yang L, Zhang C. Quercetin affects shoaling and anxiety behaviors in zebrafish: Involvement of neuroinflammation and neuron apoptosis. Fish Shellfish Immunol 2020; 105: 359-68.
[http://dx.doi.org/10.1016/j.fsi.2020.06.058] [PMID: 32693159]

CHAPTER 6

Animal Models of Zebrafish

Romanpreet Kaur[1] and **Shamsher Singh**[1,*]

[1] *Neuropharmacology Division, Department of Pharmacology, ISF College of Pharmacy, Moga, Punjab 142001, India*

INTRODUCTION

Zebrafish, scientifically known as *Danio rerio*, are small-bodied tropical, freshwater fish species originally from the rivers and streams of South Asia. They serve as a critical model organism in scientific research, particularly in the domains of genetics, developmental biology, toxicology, pharmacology, and neuroscience. Due to their extensive genetic homology to humans, Zebrafish has emerged as a widely utilized organism in biomedical and environmental studies, offering valuable insights into gene function, developmental processes, and disease mechanisms.

WHY ZEBRAFISH IS PREFERRED AS AN ANIMAL MODEL?

Zebrafish are popular species in biological research due to their diverse applications across various scientific disciplines. Despite their phylogenetic divergence from humans, Zebrafish exhibit several behavioral similarities to humans. These include complex social behaviors such as shoaling and courtship displays, as well as responses to environmental stimuli, including light and temperature variations. Additionally, Zebrafish demonstrate cognitive functions such as learning and memory formation. Notably, Zebrafish also shares analogous stress responses, reward system mechanisms, and patterns of social interaction, making it a valuable model for studying human behavior and neurobiology.

Additionally, Zebrafish and humans share several conserved molecular pathways and signaling networks that regulate essential physiological processes, including cell division, growth, and apoptosis (programmed cell death). Genomic analyses reveal that approximately 70% of human genes possess at least one identifiable homolog in Zebrafish, underscoring the significant genetic similarities between humans and Zebrafish.

[*] **Corresponding author Shamsher Singh:** Neuropharmacology Division, Department of Pharmacology, ISF College of Pharmacy, Moga, Punjab 142001, India; Tel: +91-9779980588; E-mail: shamshersinghbajwa@gmail.com

Zebrafish are the perfect model organism for genetic and developmental research due to their prolific reproduction and transparency of embryonic stages. Key advantages include:

1. Rapid embryonic development allows for efficient and accelerated research.
2. Low cost, high reproductive output, ease of genetic manipulation, and a simplified genome, facilitate experimental studies.
3. As a vertebrate, Zebrafish exhibits significant anatomical, genetic, and physiological similarities to humans, enhancing its relevance in biomedical research.
4. Tolerance to a broad range of environmental conditions, reflecting the species' natural habitat and enabling diverse experimental conditions.
5. Their small size and rapid developmental timeline make Zebrafish ideal for high-throughput screening of pharmacological agents and chemical compounds.

APPLICATIONS

1. **Disease modelling:** Zebrafish are used as a model organism for studying a range of human diseases, including cancer, mental, and neurological disorders, as well as developmental, and metabolic abnormalities. The specific areas of study in Zebrafish are described in Table **6.1**.
2. **Therapeutic compound screening:** Zebrafish are utilized in drug discovery and therapeutic compound screening processes to find possible treatments for human diseases.
3. **Environmental toxicology:** The impact of environmental pollutants on development and health can be studied using Zebrafish as a model to assess toxicological effects.
4. **Behavioural neuroscience:** Zebrafish are used in behavioural neuroscience research to explore the neuronal mechanisms underlying behaviour and cognition [1].

SCOPE OF ZEBRAFISH

Zebrafish research covers a wide range of scopes. The scope of Zebrafish in research is described in Fig. (**6.1**).

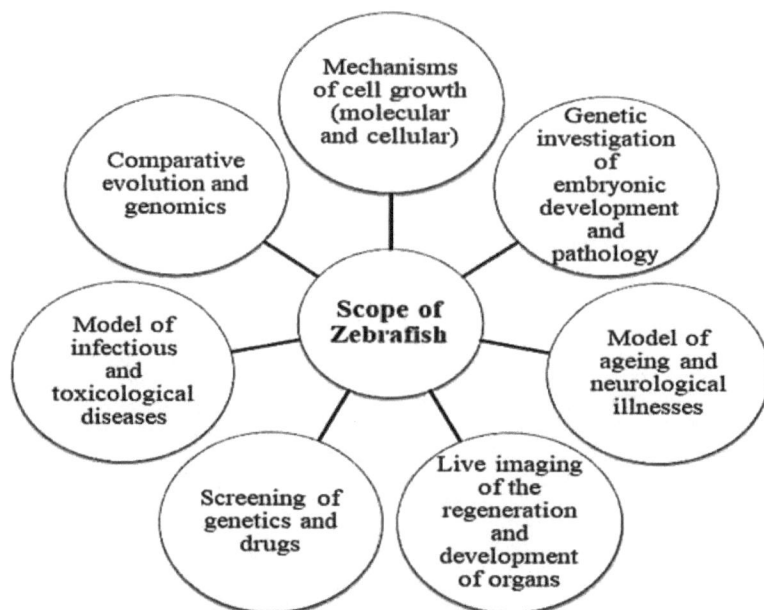

Fig. (6.1). Scope of Zebrafish.

Table 6.1. Specific areas of study in Zebrafish.

S. No.	System	Target Area
1.	Nervous System	Alzheimer's Disease, Parkinson's Disease, Amyotrophic Lateral Sclerosis (ALS), Huntington's Disease, Autism Spectrum Disorders
2.	Cardiovascular	Atrial Fibrillation, Heart Failure, Atherosclerosis, Hypertension
3.	Endocrine System	Thyroid disease, Diabetes, Cushing's disease, Obesity, Adrenal insufficiency, Nonalcoholic fatty liver disease
4.	Excretory System	Polycystic kidney disease, Ciliopathy- associated human cystic kidney diseases, Acute kidney injury
5.	Regeneration Study	Kidney, Heart, Spinal cord, Retina, Telencephalon regeneration
6.	Toxicology	Digestive system, Liver, Brain, Heart, Kidney

As a vertebrate model organism, Zebrafish are generally appealing and hold considerable potential for biomedical research and the study of human diseases.

Classification of Diseases in which Zebrafish are used as an Animal Model

Zebrafish are utilized in laboratory settings to model a wide variety of human diseases, including neurological, cardiovascular, renal, and metabolic disorders such as diabetes, digestive system diseases, cancer, and musculoskeletal conditions. These Zebrafish models provide valuable insights into the pathophysiology and potential therapeutic interventions for these ailments. The classification of diseases in which Zebrafish are used as an animal model is described in Fig. (**6.2**).

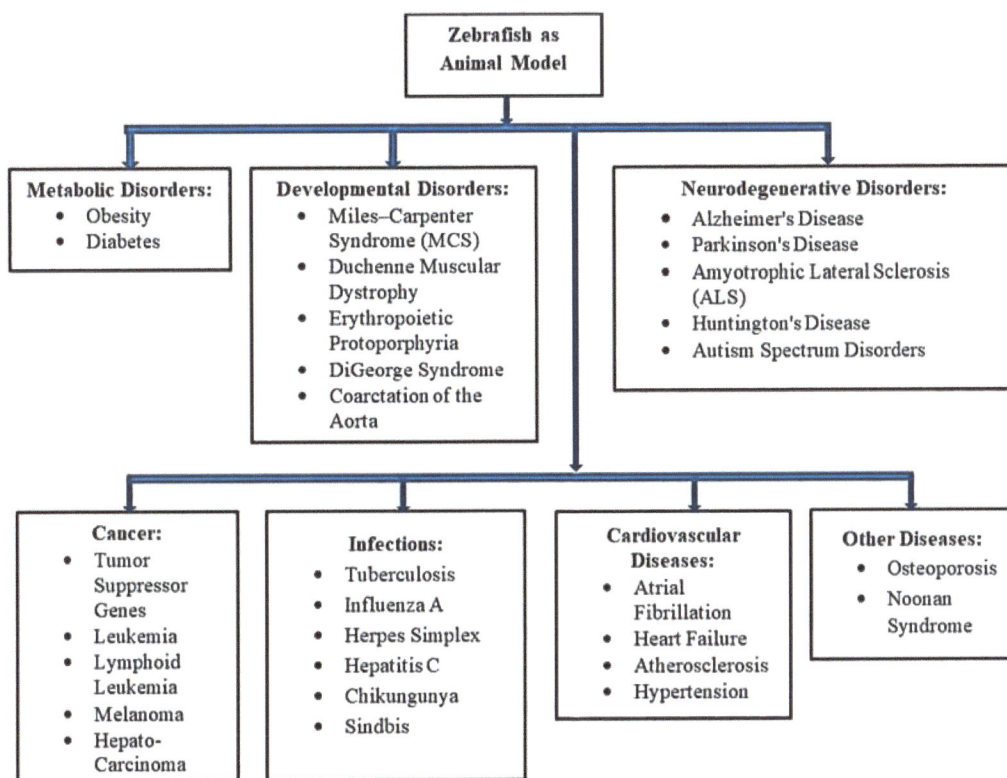

Fig. (6.2). Classification of diseases in which Zebrafish are used as an animal model.

Various methodologies, including genetic engineering, mutagenesis, and transgenesis, are employed to model these disorders in Zebrafish. These techniques enable the investigation of the underlying mechanisms of disease pathogenesis as well as the evaluation of potential therapeutic interventions [2, 3].

Metabolic Disorders

Obesity

Zebrafish share numerous physiological and metabolic characteristics with mammals, making them an excellent model for studying obesity and associated metabolic disorders. They are useful for investigating obesity in both adult and larval stages because they contain adipose tissue that is distributed and formed similarly to that of mammals. Zebrafish exhibit comparable lipid metabolism, adipogenic pathways, and metabolism-related functions, including insulin regulation, lipid storage, and appetite control. Zebrafish can be used to identify novel molecular targets for the prevention and management of obesity in humans. For instance, they are employed to investigate the regulatory molecules that control the expression of genes involved in lipid metabolism, which is dysregulated in obesity in both mammals and Zebrafish.

Diabetes

Zebrafish serve as a highly relevant and advantageous model for studying diabetes, owing to their significant physiological similarities to mammals, particularly in glucose metabolism and vascular development. Zebrafish are particularly useful for modeling type 2 diabetes mellitus (T2DM), as they exhibit a rapid onset of T2DM-like symptoms and respond to anti-diabetic treatments in a manner analogous to humans. Additionally, the Zebrafish transcriptome closely mirrors that of humans with T2DM, enabling the identification of pathophysiological pathways and providing a robust platform for investigating the molecular mechanisms of the disease and testing potential therapeutic interventions [4].

Developmental Disorders

Miles-Carpenter Syndrome (MCS)

Miles-Carpenter Syndrome (MCS) is a rare hereditary disorder characterized by craniofacial deformities, intellectual impairment, and developmental delays. Zebrafish are suitable for genetic manipulation techniques such as CRISPR/Cas9, which allow for the introduction of specific mutations analogous to those found in human genetic disorders. Using this method has made it possible to mimic several genetic disorders that have an impact on craniofacial development and to investigate the underlying genetic pathways of MCS.

Duchenne Muscular Dystrophy

Zebrafish are used to model Duchenne muscular dystrophy (DMD), a severe type of disease that is characterized by gradual muscle weakness and degradation. Zebrafish models of DMD have several advantages over other animal models for preclinical research as Zebrafish models mimic the severity of symptoms seen in human DMD and it is also easier to assess skeletal and cardiac muscle phenotypes (structure and function), as well as other biomarkers.

Erythropoietin Protoporphyria

Erythropoietic protoporphyria (EPP) is a rare genetic disorder that disrupts heme biosynthesis, leading to the accumulation of protoporphyrin IX in the body. They serve as an effective model for studying EPP due to its conserved mechanisms of erythropoiesis, which are regulated both extrinsically by erythropoietin secreted from adjacent tissues and organs, and intrinsically by transcription factors expressed in erythroid cells. This makes Zebrafish a valuable organism for investigating the pathophysiology of EPP and for exploring potential therapeutic interventions targeting the dysregulated heme synthesis pathway.

DiGeorge Syndrome

Zebrafish are used to represent DiGeorge syndrome also known as 22q11.2 deletion syndrome, a chromosomal condition that causes multiple body systems to develop poorly. Heart problems weakened immune systems, cleft palates, and low blood calcium levels can all be caused by the condition. Humans and Zebrafish share a large amount of DNA, including several genes that are syntenic to human chromosome 22q11.2, the location of the microdeletion linked to DGS. Because of its genetic closeness, researchers can use genome editing methods such as CRISPR/Cas9 to generate similar deletions in Zebrafish embryos, allowing them to examine certain genetic pathways causing DGS.

Coarctation of the Aorta

Coarctation of the aorta is a congenital cardiac defect characterized by the narrowing or constriction of the aorta. Zebrafish harboring the "gridlock" gene mutation (grlm145) exhibit aortic dysmorphogenesis that closely resembles congenital aortic coarctation in humans. This mutation results in the absence of circulation in the trunk and tail, providing a relevant model for studying the pathophysiology of aortic coarctation and offering insights into the genetic and developmental mechanisms underlying this congenital cardiovascular abnormality [5].

Neurodegenerative Disorders

Alzheimer's Disease

Zebrafish are used to model Alzheimer's disease, which is characterized by the buildup of beta-amyloid plaques and neurofibrillary tangles in the brain. Zebrafish and humans are highly similar in terms of genetics and molecular makeup, with numerous orthologs linked to neurodegenerative illnesses like Alzheimer's. To understand the disease causes, this enables the development of Zebrafish models with mutations in genes connected to human AD.

Parkinson's Disease

Zebrafish are used to model Parkinson's disease, which is characterized by the loss of dopamine-producing neurons in the substantia nigra. The dopaminergic system in Zebrafish is similar to humans. Zebrafish and humans share many brain structures and dopaminergic circuits, making it easier to study how dopamine function abnormalities affect PD symptoms.

Amyotrophic Lateral Sclerosis (ALS)

Zebrafish are utilized as a model organism for amyotrophic lateral sclerosis (ALS), a neurodegenerative disorder characterized by the progressive degeneration of motor neurons in the spinal cord and brain. Zebrafish models effectively replicate the cellular and behavioral phenotypes associated with ALS, offering valuable insights into the pathophysiology and potential diagnostic markers of the disease. Furthermore, these models facilitate the identification and evaluation of therapeutic strategies, providing a robust platform for discovering novel treatments for ALS.

Huntington's Disease

Huntington's disease models in Zebrafish effectively replicate key aspects of human neurodegeneration, including the progressive loss of neurons, particularly within regions such as the striatum, which are central to the disease. This provides an invaluable platform for investigating the underlying mechanisms of neuronal dysfunction and degeneration, enabling researchers to explore the molecular and cellular processes contributing to the pathophysiology of Huntington's disease and to identify potential therapeutic targets.

Autism Spectrum Disorders

Zebrafish are increasingly utilized as a model organism to study autism spectrum disorders (ASD), a group of neurodevelopmental conditions characterized by deficits in social interaction, communication, and repetitive behaviors. Zebrafish possess orthologous genes that are implicated in ASD, allowing for the targeted mutation of these genes in a manner that closely parallels human ASD pathophysiology. This genetic similarity enables the modeling of ASD-related traits in Zebrafish, providing valuable insights into the molecular and behavioral mechanisms underlying these disorders and facilitating the development of potential therapeutic interventions [6].

Cancer

Tumor Suppressor Genes (e.g., p53 and apc)

Zebrafish are extensively used to investigate the role of tumor suppressor genes in cancer development and progression. The Zebrafish p53 tumor suppressor gene shares a high degree of homology with its mammalian counterpart, making it an effective model for studying the function of p53 in oncogenesis. Zebrafish research has elucidated the critical role of p53 mutations in the development of various tumor types and has contributed to the identification of novel regulatory mechanisms that may underlie the disruption of the p53 pathway in human cancers. Additionally, Zebrafish with the APC+/ genotype spontaneously develop liver tumors, and transcriptomic analyses comparing Zebrafish and human liver tumors have revealed a remarkable conservation of molecular signatures and tumor progression patterns, further establishing Zebrafish as a relevant model for cancer research.

Leukaemia

Zebrafish serve as a valuable model for leukemia, a malignancy characterized by the uncontrolled growth and proliferation of white blood cells. The hematopoietic system in Zebrafish exhibits a high degree of similarity to that of humans, with many aspects of hematopoiesis, the process of blood cell formation, being conserved. This similarity makes Zebrafish an excellent model for studying the initiation, progression, and dissemination of leukemia, offering key insights into the molecular and cellular mechanisms underlying this form of malignancy.

Lymphoid Leukaemia

The Zebrafish model is a valuable tool for understanding lymphoid leukemia, a cancer characterized by the abnormal proliferation and development of lymphoid cells. The blood cells of Zebrafish share conserved genetic pathways associated with leukemia and exhibit molecular similarities to human blood cells, making them an ideal model for studying the disease. In one study, Zebrafish expressing the TEL-AML1 fusion gene exhibited lethal lymphoid hyperplasia as early as 28 days post-fertilization, with approximately 6% of the fish affected. This model provides important insights into the molecular mechanisms underlying lymphoid leukemia and facilitates the exploration of potential therapeutic strategies.

Melanoma

Zebrafish serve as a relevant model for studying melanoma, a type of skin cancer. Melanocytes, the pigment-producing cells responsible for melanomas in humans, are also present in Zebrafish, making them an effective system for melanoma research. The crestin gene in Zebrafish, which is expressed in neural crest progenitors (NCPs) during development and repressed in melanoma tumors, serves as a valuable marker for tracking melanoma progression. This model provides significant insights into the molecular mechanisms underlying melanoma pathogenesis and offers a platform for evaluating potential therapeutic interventions.

Hepato-carcinoma

Zebrafish are increasingly utilized as a model for studying hepatocellular carcinoma (HCC), a form of liver cancer. The liver structure of Zebrafish closely resembles that of mammals, featuring polarized hepatocytes organized within a complex microenvironment composed of biliary epithelial cells, liver sinusoidal endothelial cells (LSECs), hepatic stellate cells (HSCs), and various immune cell types. Furthermore, the development of hepatocellular carcinoma in Zebrafish livers closely mirrors the histological features observed in mammalian systems, making Zebrafish an invaluable model for investigating the molecular mechanisms of liver cancer and for testing potential therapeutic strategies [7].

Infections

Tuberculosis

Zebrafish are widely recognized as a preferred animal model for studying tuberculosis, a bacterial infection caused by *Mycobacterium tuberculosis*. Zebrafish are particularly sensitive to *Mycobacterium marinum*, a naturally occurring fish pathogen that induces a condition resembling tuberculosis in cold-blooded vertebrates. This susceptibility makes Zebrafish an excellent model for investigating the pathogenesis of tuberculosis, host-pathogen interactions, and the immune response, providing valuable insights into the molecular mechanisms underlying the disease and potential therapeutic strategies.

Influenza A

The Zebrafish model has a profound impact on the study of influenza A, a viral infection caused by the Influenza A virus (IAV). This model allows for the detailed investigation of both innate and adaptive immune responses in Zebrafish in the context of viral infections, including influenza A. Strains of Influenza A virus that target the respiratory epithelium of Zebrafish can induce infections that closely resemble human respiratory infections, providing an effective *in vivo* system for studying viral pathogenesis, host immune responses, and potential therapeutic interventions for influenza A.

Herpes Simplex

Zebrafish are extensively employed as a model organism for studying herpes simplex virus (HSV) infections, particularly those caused by Herpes simplex virus type 1 (HSV-1). Zebrafish provide a valuable *in vivo* system for investigating the pathogenesis of HSV-1, especially its effects on the neurological system. Their transparent embryos, coupled with advanced imaging techniques, enable real-time, high-resolution analysis of viral propagation and host-virus interactions, making them an indispensable tool for elucidating the molecular mechanisms underlying HSV-1 infections and for developing potential therapeutic strategies.

Hepatitis C

Zebrafish are preferred as a model organism for studying hepatitis C, a viral infection caused by the Hepatitis C virus (HCV). Zebrafish are capable of replicating HCV sub-replicons and expressing HCV-related proteins within their livers, making them an effective system for investigating the molecular mechanisms of HCV replication and pathogenesis. This model offers valuable insights into transcriptional modifications of host genes, liver disease progression, and viral replication dynamics. Furthermore, Zebrafish can be employed in the screening and evaluation of anti-HCV therapeutics, providing a robust platform for drug discovery and development.

Chikungunya

Zebrafish are used as a model organism to investigate the pathogenesis of chikungunya, a viral infection caused by Chikungunya virus (CHIKV). Zebrafish offer the advantage of real-time, high-resolution observation of viral behavior and propagation at the cellular level, enabling detailed analysis of the viral life cycle and host interactions. This model is invaluable for elucidating the molecular mechanisms underlying CHIKV pathogenesis and for the development of effective vaccines and therapeutic interventions.

Sindbis

Zebrafish serve as a model organism for studying the pathogenesis of Sindbis virus (SINV) infection. Sindbis virus is an arboviral pathogen that causes a range of clinical manifestations. They are particularly well-suited for modeling SINV due to their ability to display the virus's multiple routes of entry and its interactions with the host's immune system, providing valuable insights into the mechanisms of viral infection and host-pathogen dynamics [8].

Cardiovascular Diseases

Atrial Fibrillation

Deregulation of the PITX2c gene, which is implicated in atrial fibrillation (AF), is associated with abnormal atrial rhythm and an increased heart rate. Mutations in Zebrafish that result in the loss of function of the PITX2c gene exhibit several phenotypic traits that are characteristic of human AF, thereby establishing Zebrafish as a valuable model for studying the pathophysiology of atrial fibrillation.

Heart Dailure

Zebrafish serve as an invaluable model for studying heart failure due to their tolerance to blood flow defects, optical transparency, and the ability to survive for extended periods without a functional circulatory system. The anatomical and physiological similarities of the Zebrafish heart to that of mammals, combined with its rapid and relatively accessible development and the availability of advanced genetic tools, position Zebrafish as a promising model for investigating human cardiac pathologies and exploring potential therapeutic approaches.

Atherosclerosis

Zebrafish are utilized as a model to investigate the progression of atherosclerosis, a condition characterized by the accumulation of lipid-rich plaques in the arterial walls. A cholesterol-enriched diet induces the formation of atherosclerotic plaques in Zebrafish, which closely resemble the early stages of atherosclerosis observed in humans. Furthermore, Zebrafish embryos exhibit additional features relevant to the disease, such as impaired vascular regeneration and repair, making them an effective *in vivo* system for studying the molecular mechanisms underlying atherosclerosis and evaluating potential therapeutic interventions.

Hypertension

Zebrafish and humans share significant similarities in their cardiovascular systems, rendering Zebrafish a valuable model organism for studying hypertension. The heart rate of Zebrafish more closely resembles that of humans than that of mice, and its electrocardiogram (ECG) patterns exhibit notable similarities to human ECG profiles. These parallels make Zebrafish an effective model for investigating the pathophysiology of cardiovascular diseases, including hypertension [9].

Other Diseases

Osteoporosis

Zebrafish have been preferred as a model for osteoporosis studies due to the presence of specific mutants and transgenic insertion mutants that exhibit altered bone mineralization. Also, Zebrafish's bones are made of collagen and calcium phosphate, just like human bones, making Zebrafish a suitable model to research bone mineralization and metabolism. This similarity enables the study of bone development, homeostasis, and pathological conditions.

Noonan Syndrome

Noonan syndrome is a rare genetic disorder associated with developmental abnormalities and intellectual disability. Research has yielded valuable insights into the pathophysiology of this condition. Zebrafish models harboring mutations in the lztr1 gene, implicated in Noonan syndrome, were generated using CRISPR-Cas9 genome editing. Ventricular hypertrophy, a feature of cardiomyopathy linked to Noonan syndrome, was discovered through histological examinations of Zebrafish.

DRUG ADMINISTRATION IN ZEBRAFISH

A range of methodologies are employed to administer pharmacological substances to Zebrafish for research purposes. Key considerations in the administration of drugs to Zebrafish include the following:

Methods of Drug Administration

1. **Water-soluble compounds:** The direct introduction of water-soluble chemicals into the aquatic environment of Zebrafish presents significant challenges for long-term pharmacological treatments, as the final concentration of the drug absorbed by the fish remains difficult to quantify, potentially leading to variability in therapeutic outcomes.
2. **Food-based drug pellets:** Food-based medicated pellets offer a non-invasive method for administering drugs to adult Zebrafish. This approach is particularly suitable for long-term therapeutic regimens, as it ensures precise dosage control and minimizes animal stress.
3. **Oral gavage and injection:** Oral gavage and injectable methods provide more accurate dosing than water-based delivery; however, they are invasive, carry risks of morbidity or mortality, and necessitate repeated anesthesia, raising concerns regarding animal welfare and the ethical implications of their use.

4. **Spawning insects:** Spawning inserts enable the transfer of groups of fish into a medicated solution, allowing for precise and controlled dosing of each individual within the group. This method offers a non-invasive means of drug administration while maintaining accurate dosage across multiple subjects [10].

ADVANTAGES

1. **Non-invasive:** Non-invasive methodologies, such as spawning inserts and food-based medicated pellets, minimize fish discomfort and stress, thereby enhancing the welfare of the organism during experimental procedures.
2. **Precise dosing:** These non-invasive methods allow for accurate control over the dosage of medication administered to each individual fish, ensuring consistent and reliable treatment delivery.
3. **Long-term treatments:** They work well for long-term medication regimens, which are crucial for researching the impacts of repeated drug exposure [11].

LIMITATIONS

1. **Water soluble compounds:** The direct addition of water-soluble substances to the aquatic environment of Zebrafish may lead to the absorption of compounds by the fish at unquantified concentrations, potentially confounding experimental outcomes and complicating dose-response assessments.
2. **Invasive methods:** Techniques such as oral gavage and injection represent invasive procedures that, while useful for the precise administration of substances, carry inherent risks of morbidity and mortality, raising ethical concerns regarding animal welfare and the potential for unintended harm.

FUTURE DIRECTIONS

1. **Gene editing:** The application of gene editing techniques, such as CRISPR-Cas9, enables more precise modeling of human diseases by introducing specific mutations or gene knockouts in Zebrafish. This facilitates the investigation of disease mechanisms and the functional role of individual genes in pathogenesis.
2. **Microbiome research:** The use of Zebrafish in microbiome research offers valuable insights into the microbiome's impact on development and health. This model provides a platform for exploring the microbiome's contributions to human disorders, elucidating its role in disease onset and progression [12].

CONCLUSION

Zebrafish are highly valuable model organisms across diverse areas of biological research. Their distinctive characteristics, including external fertilization and transparent embryos, render them particularly suitable for studies in developmental biology, physiology, and genetics. Since Zebrafish and humans share a great deal of functional conservation in their morphology, genetics, and physiology. Zebrafish has become a widely used model for investigating a broad range of human diseases and for the development of potential therapeutic interventions.

PRACTICE QUESTIONS

1. In which disease Zebrafish are used as a model?
2. What are the drug administration processes in Zebrafish?
3. In which neurological disorders were Zebrafish used as a model?
4. Which apparatus is used to perform practicals in Zebrafish?
5. Give a brief description of why Zebrafish are used as a model?

REFERENCES

[1]   MacRae CA, Peterson RT. Zebrafish as a mainstream model for *in vivo* systems pharmacology and toxicology. Annu Rev Pharmacol Toxicol 2023; 63(1): 43-64.
        [http://dx.doi.org/10.1146/annurev-pharmtox-051421-105617] [PMID: 36151053]

[2]   Filik N, Vital A. Vital A fish: A critical review of Zebrafish models in disease scenario and case reports screens. Laboratuvar Hayvanları Bilimi ve Uygulamaları Dergisi 2024; 4(2): 53-9.
        [http://dx.doi.org/10.62425/jlasp.1426010]

[3]   Burgess HA, Burton EA. A critical review of Zebrafish neurological disease models−1. The premise: Neuroanatomical, cellular and genetic homology and experimental tractability. Oxf Open Neurosci 2023; 2: kvac018.
        [http://dx.doi.org/10.1093/oons/kvac018] [PMID: 37649777]

[4]   Ghaddar B, Diotel N. Zebrafish: A new promise to study the impact of metabolic disorders on the brain. Int J Mol Sci 2022; 23(10): 5372.
        [http://dx.doi.org/10.3390/ijms23105372] [PMID: 35628176]

[5]   de Abreu MS, Genario R, Giacomini ACVV, *et al.* Zebrafish as a model of neurodevelopmental disorders. Neuroscience 2020; 445: 3-11.
        [http://dx.doi.org/10.1016/j.neuroscience.2019.08.034] [PMID: 31472215]

[6]   Chia K, Klingseisen A, Sieger D, Priller J. Zebrafish as a model organism for neurodegenerative disease. Front Mol Neurosci 2022; 15: 940484.
        [http://dx.doi.org/10.3389/fnmol.2022.940484] [PMID: 36311026]

[7]   Mione MC, Trede NS. The Zebrafish as a model for cancer. Dis Model Mech 2010; 3(9-10): 517-23.
        [http://dx.doi.org/10.1242/dmm.004747] [PMID: 20354112]

[8]   Novoa B, Figueras A. Zebrafish: model for the study of inflammation and the innate immune response to infectious diseases. Current topics in innate immunity II. 2012: 253-75.
        [http://dx.doi.org/10.1007/978-1-4614-0106-3_15]

[9]   Bournele D, Beis D. Zebrafish models of cardiovascular disease. Heart Fail Rev 2016; 21(6): 803-13.
        [http://dx.doi.org/10.1007/s10741-016-9579-y] [PMID: 27503203]

[10]   Chaoul V, Dib EY, Bedran J, *et al.* Assessing drug administration techniques in Zebrafish models of neurological disease. Int J Mol Sci 2023; 24(19): 14898.
        [http://dx.doi.org/10.3390/ijms241914898] [PMID: 37834345]

[11]   Gerlai R. Zebrafish (*Danio rerio*): A newcomer with great promise in behavioral neuroscience. Neurosci Biobehav Rev 2023; 144: 104978.
        [http://dx.doi.org/10.1016/j.neubiorev.2022.104978] [PMID: 36442644]

[12]   Simonetti RB, Marques LS, Streit DP Jr, Oberst ER. Zebrafish (*Danio rerio*): The future of animal model in biomedical research. J FisheriesSciences Com 2015; 9(3): 39.

CHAPTER 7

Novel Tank Diving Test in Zebrafish

Falguni Goel[1], Romanpreet Kaur[1], Vaishali[1] and Shamsher Singh[1,*]

[1] *Neuropharmacology Division, Department of Pharmacology, ISF College of Pharmacy, Moga, Punjab 142001, India*

INTRODUCTION

Aim: To check for anxiety in adult Zebrafish by using a novel diving test.

Scope and outcomes: We would be able to know about the anxiety-like behavior in Zebrafish by this practical. A novel diving test is an apparatus that is wide from top and narrow from bottom. The top zone shows that the fish is active, and the bottom zone shows that the fish is anxious. Researchers observe and record their behavior, including diving depth, duration underwater, and swimming patterns.

Theory: A novel diving test in Zebrafish could be designed to assess their behavioral responses (anxiety) and physiological adaptations to underwater conditions [1]. A novel diving test is an innovative method to test anxiety by moving the fish (by net) to a unique tank for behavioral observation as well as phenotyping, Zebrafish are subjected to research testing in an initial treatment beaker. Using a beaker used for pre-treatment, groups of controls go through identical steps without interruption. The measurement of the tank is $60 \times 30 \times 46$ cm (length × width × height). The novel diving test apparatus is shown in Fig. (7.1).

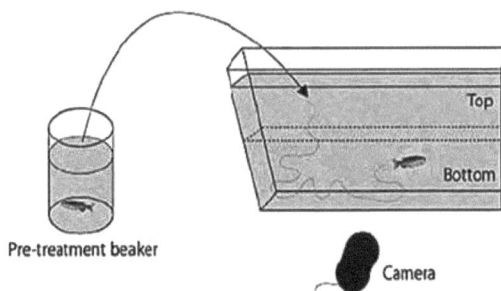

Fig. (7.1). Diagram illustrating the mechanism of the novel diving test.

* **Corresponding author Shamsher Singh:** Neuropharmacology Division, Department of Pharmacology, ISF College of Pharmacy, Moga, Punjab 142001, India; Tel: +91-9779980588; E-mail: shamshersinghbajwa@gmail.com

REQUIREMENTS

Animal: Adult Zebrafish

Equipment: Novel Tank Diving apparatus, Any-maze software, Graph pad prism, Camera.

PROCEDURE

1. Firstly, take one healthy Zebrafish for the procedure.
2. Move it to the Novel diving apparatus with the help of a net.
3. Now make sure that there is no noise while following the procedure.
4. Leave the fish for 10 minutes in the tank for habituation.
5. Now place the camera to record the video and analyse it for 10 minutes.
6. If the fish spends more time in the bottom zone then it is showing anxiety-like symptoms.

Parameters Measured

1. **Diving depth:** The maximum depth reached by each Zebrafish during the test period could be measured using depth sensors or video tracking systems.
2. **Duration underwater:** The amount of time spent by each Zebrafish submerged could be recorded to assess their ability to stay underwater.
3. **Swimming patterns:** Researchers could analyse the swimming patterns of Zebrafish while diving, including speed, directionality, and any deviations from typical behaviour [1].

Physiological measurements: In addition to behavioral observations, physiological parameters such as oxygen consumption, heart rate, and metabolic rate could be measured to assess the physiological adaptations of Zebrafish to underwater diving.

Experimental conditions: The diving test could be conducted under various experimental conditions to study the effects of factors such as water temperature, oxygen levels, and environmental stressors on Zebrafish diving behavior and physiology.

Data analysis: Data collected from the diving test could be analyzed using statistical methods to identify patterns and correlations between behavioral responses, physiological parameters, and experimental conditions.

OBSERVATION

A dummy analysis is given in Table **7.1**.

Table 7.1. Observation table of number of entry and time spent in top and bottom zones on the novel tank diving test apparatus of Zebrafish.

S. No.	Time Spent in the Top Zone (sec)	Time Spent in the Bottom Zone (sec)	No. of Entries in the Top Zone	No. of Entries in the Bottom Zone
1.	15	38	3	10
2.	10	49	3	11
3.	16	35	5	9
4.	18	41	4	10
Mean	14.75±3.4	40.75±6.0	3.75±0.9	10±0.8

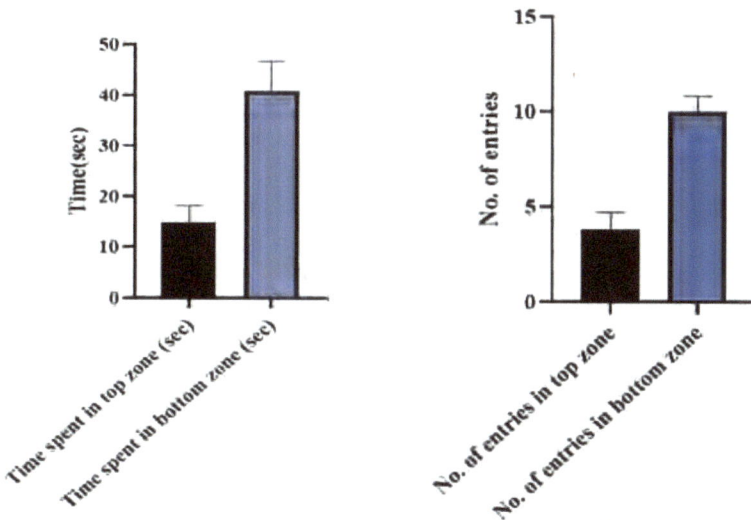

Statistical analysis: Statistical analysis indicates that the time spent and the number of entries in the top zone have decreased, while the time spent and the number of entries in the bottom zone have increased.

RESULT

The novel diving test was performed, and the time was recorded successfully. The results have shown that the time spent and the number of entries in the top zone have decreased, while the time spent and the number of entries in the bottom zone have increased.

APPLICATIONS

1. **Anxiety assessment:** The test provides a valuable tool for assessing anxiety levels in Zebrafish by monitoring behavioral responses in unfamiliar

environments, offering critical insights into their coping mechanisms and emotional states.

2. **Pharmacological studies:** This assay is instrumental in evaluating the effects of anxiogenic and anxiolytic compounds, contributing to the development of novel therapeutic strategies for anxiety and stress-related disorders.

3. **Genetic research:** By utilizing this test, researchers can compare different Zebrafish strains, facilitating the investigation of the genetic underpinnings of anxiety-related behaviors and contributing to the understanding of genetic factors influencing emotional regulation.

4. **Neurodevelopmental studies:** The test serves as a useful model for assessing how environmental stressors, such as exposure to pollutants or other neurodevelopmental disruptors, impact behavior and brain development, thereby aiding in the study of environmental influences on neurodevelopment.

5. **Behavioural ecology:** This test provides insight into the behavioral ecology of Zebrafish, allowing researchers to investigate how these fish adjust their behavior in response to novel or potentially threatening environments, thus enhancing our understanding of survival strategies in naturalistic contexts.

6. **Comparative studies:** The test can be employed across multiple fish species to examine anxiety-related behaviors, thus broadening our understanding of evolutionary adaptations and the comparative aspects of stress responses across diverse taxa.

7. **Longitudinal studies:** By enabling the monitoring of behavioral changes over time, this test proves valuable for longitudinal studies focused on aging, developmental processes, and the long-term effects of environmental or pharmacological interventions on behaviour [2].

ADVANTAGES

1. **Stress and anxiety assessment:** The test provides a precise evaluation of stress and anxiety levels in animals. Upon exposure to novel environments, the diving behavior, a natural escape response, can serve as an indicator of the animal's anxiety levels, offering valuable insights into its emotional state.

2. **Naturalistic behaviour:** Unlike other behavioural tests that may need significant training or entail artificial circumstances, the innovative diving test makes use of the animals' innate behaviour, resulting in more accurate and valid findings.

3. **Minimal training required:** The test typically does not necessitate substantial training or conditioning of the animal, which minimizes time investment and reduces the risk of confounding variables associated with training processes.

4. **Ethological relevance:** The test is ethically relevant since it simulates a realistic escape reaction. This makes the data more useful for understanding

natural behaviour and their underlying causes as compared to mammalian models.

5. **Measurable data:** It gives unambiguous, measurable data such as dive delay, dive frequency, and time spent in an unfamiliar environment, which may be utilized to diagnose anxiety and stress.

6. **Sensitive to pharmacological manipulation:** Because the test is sensitive to both anxiolytic and anxiogenic medication treatments, it may be used to assess the effects of pharmacological agents on anxiety and stress reactions.

7. **Non-invasive:** As a non-invasive procedure, the test minimizes the risk of physical harm or undue stress that could confound the results, ensuring the integrity of the behavioral data collected.

8. **Broad applicability:** The test is adaptable to a wide range of species, particularly rodents, allowing for comparative studies of anxiety and stress responses across different animal models, enhancing its utility in diverse research contexts.

9. **High throughput:** The test is compatible with high-throughput protocols, enabling the rapid assessment of multiple animals in a short time frame. This is particularly advantageous for studies involving large sample sizes or for screening purposes.

10. **Behavioural insights:** It may provide light on other areas of behaviour, such as exploratory behaviour and coping mechanisms, which are important for understanding the animal's entire behavioural phenotype [3].

LIMITATIONS

1. **Species-specific behaviour:** The test may not be appropriate for other animals or provide significant findings for those of other species, since it is mainly designed for rats. It is possible that not all species display the behaviour under study in the same manner.

2. **Environmental conditions:** Several environmental conditions, including temperature, noise level, and illumination, might affect results. These elements must be properly managed to guarantee data consistency and dependability.

3. **Restricted Scope:** Although the exam assesses behaviour linked to stress and anxiety, it could not provide a thorough understanding of other facets of cognitive or mental health. It might take further examinations to get a full behavioural profile.

4. **Effects of habituation:** Repeated exposure of an animal to the test environment may lead to habituation, potentially diminishing the test's sensitivity to anxiety across multiple trials. This could compromise the validity of repeated measurements of anxiety.

5. **Physical condition of animals:** The physical condition of the animals, including their swimming capabilities and overall health, can influence their

performance in the test. Animals with physical impairments may not exhibit the expected diving behavior, potentially introducing bias or confounding factors into the results.

6. **Training and handling:** Although minimal training is necessary, handling the animal prior to the test can affect its stress levels and subsequent behaviour during the test. Variability in handling procedures may introduce inconsistencies, thereby influencing the reliability of the data obtained [3].

PRACTICE QUESTIONS

1. What is the measurement of the Novel diving test?
2. Why is it called a novel diving test?
3. Why it is narrow from the bottom?
4. Why is a novel diving test performed?
5. What is the alternative to the novel diving test?

REFERENCES

[1]   Muralidharan A, Swaminathan A, Poulose A. Deep learning dives: Predicting anxiety in zebrafish through novel tank assay analysis. Physiol Behav 2024; 287114696
[http://dx.doi.org/10.1016/j.physbeh.2024.114696] [PMID: 39293590]

[2]   Fitzgerald JA, Könemann S, Krümpelmann L, Županič A, vom Berg C. Approaches to test the neurotoxicity of environmental contaminants in the zebrafish model: From behavior to molecular mechanisms. Environ Toxicol Chem 2020; 40(4): 989-1006.
[http://dx.doi.org/10.1002/etc.4951] [PMID: 33270929]

[3]   Vaz R, Hofmeister W, Lindstrand A. Zebrafish models of neurodevelopmental disorders: limitations and benefits of current tools and techniques. Int J Mol Sci 2019; 20(6): 1296.
[http://dx.doi.org/10.3390/ijms20061296] [PMID: 30875831]

CHAPTER 8

Social Preference Test in Zebrafish

Falguni Goel[1]**, Mayank Attri**[1]**, Khadga Raj**[1] **and Shamsher Singh**[1,*]

[1] *Neuropharmacology Division, Department of Pharmacology, ISF College of Pharmacy, Moga, Punjab 142001, India*

INTRODUCTION

Aim: To study the social behavior preference test in Zebrafish (*Danio rerio*).

Scope and outcomes: The social preference test holds significant value for examining the potential translational effects of hormones, pharmaceuticals, medical interventions, and other pharmacological agents. Additionally, it serves as a critical tool for studying factors that may influence zebrafish social behavior in laboratory settings. This test offers promising utility in the development of a reliable zebrafish model for investigating various neurological disorders characterized by social deficits, as well as psychological conditions. A rectangular tank split into two compartments with a transparent barrier enabling direct vision among the experimental fishes and the shoal can be utilized to examine social interactions toward a single stimulus. The usage of a rectangular tank featuring three different areas is highly regarded for evaluating preference for two distinct social cues simultaneously.

Theory: The tendency of individuals to associate and reside near others who share similar characteristics is referred to as social preference. In Zebrafish, this social behavior is assessed by observing and analyzing the subject's responses to or interactions with a given social stimulus [1]. Similar to behavioral tests conducted on rodents, social preference tests have been developed for Zebrafish. These tests typically consist of two distinct phases to evaluate social behavior effectively [2]. The Zebrafish under scrutiny is preserved alone in a compartment of the test tank throughout the first phase, acknowledged as the habituation phase, to get accustomed to the unfamiliar surroundings. The initial introduction of the social stimulus, which usually involves the introduction of a couple of small groups of similar living species, commences the second phase, which is the interaction phase [3]. As an alternative, digitally animated (moving) visuals of

---

* **Corresponding author Shamsher Singh:** Neuropharmacology Division, Department of Pharmacology, ISF College of Pharmacy, Moga, Punjab 142001, India; Tel: +91-9779980588; E-mail: shamshersinghbajwa@gmail.com

Zebrafish, the augmented and virtual systems, or a pre-recorded film of live fish displayed on a computer screen could be used as the social stimulus [4] (Fig. **8.1**).

The social preference test remains a straightforward, accessible, and flexible method that holds the potential to offer novel insights into the mechanisms underlying neuropsychiatric and neurodevelopmental disorders characterized by impairments in social functioning. Two major benefits that may crop up by executing this test in neurobehavioral research are that contrary to the shoaling and schooling assays, the social preference test has the benefit of inspecting a single subject instead of a group of subjects [5].

Along with that, the social stimulus in the social preference test is less intimidating to those in the mirror biting and predator exposure tests, it could possibly be interpreted as a low-stress assay [6].

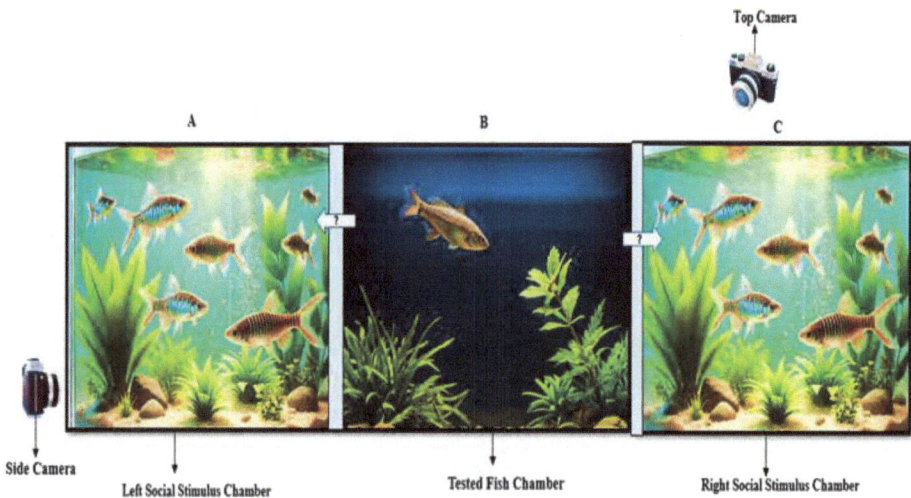

Fig. (8.1). Diagrammatic illustration for social preference test.

EXPERIMENTAL SETUP

The social preference test typically involves a tank divided into three compartments: a central chamber and two side chambers. The side chambers may either be identical or contain distinct visual cues to differentiate them.

Habituation phase: Zebrafish are first habituated to the experimental setup by allowing them to freely explore the entire tank without any social stimuli present. This phase helps acclimate the fish to the test environment.

Social preference phase: In this phase, a stimulus fish (a conspecific) is introduced into one of the side chambers, while the other side chamber remains empty or contains a non-social stimulus (*e.g.*, an object). The focal Zebrafish is then placed in the central chamber and allowed to freely interact with both the conspecific and non-social stimulus.

Behavioral observations: During the social preference phase, researchers observe and record the behavior of the focal Zebrafish. Key behavioral parameters, including the time spent in each chamber, the frequency and duration of interactions with the conspecific compared to the non-social stimulus, and specific social behaviors (*e.g.*, shoaling and courtship displays), are systematically measured.

Analysis of social preference: The preference of the focal Zebrafish for the conspecific *versus* the non-social stimulus is assessed based on the amount of time spent interacting with each stimulus and other relevant behavioral measures. An increased preference for the conspecific is indicative of social preference or sociability.

Experimental conditions: The social preference test can be conducted under different experimental conditions to investigate the effects of genetic mutations, drug treatments, environmental manipulations, or social experiences on Zebrafish social behavior. Additionally, the test can be modified to study specific aspects of social behavior, such as aggression, dominance, or social learning.

REQUIREMENTS

Animal: Adult Zebrafish

Equipment: Social preference test apparatus, ANY-maze, Camera, Graph-pad-prism.

PROCEDURE

The social performance test requires only three sessions: the habituation phase, training session, testing session

1. The optimal approach involves selecting healthy Zebrafish for the experiment, ensuring that each procedural step is conducted according to the guidelines established by the Committee for Control and Supervision of Experiments on Animals (CPCSEA).
2. Secondly, a net should be utilized for transferring the chosen Zebrafish directly into the test tank.

3. The observational results could become distorted; therefore, the researcher has to make sure that there is no noise while carrying out the experimental procedures.
4. After that, the subject (Zebrafish) ought to be given about ten minutes to get habituated to the equipment.
5. Now, set the camera to capture the video evidence, and then give another ten minutes for the researcher to assess.
6. The fish typically exhibits social activity when approaching the stimulus and social inactivity when avoiding it, leading to a logical conclusion based on these observations.

Data Analysis

Data obtained from the social preference test are subjected to statistical analysis to identify significant differences in social behavior across experimental groups or conditions. Such analyses offer valuable insights into the neural circuits, genetic determinants, and environmental factors that influence social behavior in zebrafish.

OBSERVATION

A dummy analysis is given in Table **8.1**.

Table 8.1. Observation table of time spent near and far from stimulus on the social preference test apparatus of Zebrafish.

S. No.	Time Spent Near the Stimulus (Sec)	Time Spent Far from the Stimulus (Sec)
1.	40	20
2.	60	30
3.	80	40
4.	20	60
Mean	50 ± 22.3	37.5 ± 14.7

Time spent near the stimulus (sec)

Time spent far from the stimulus (sec)

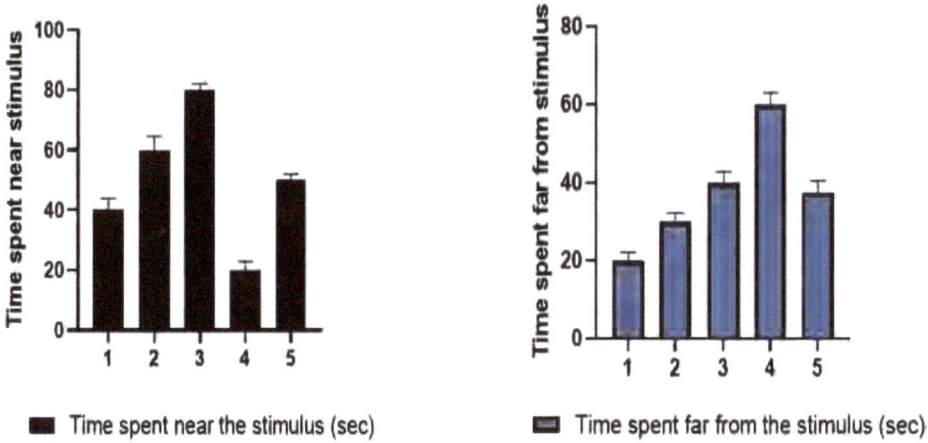

Statistical Analysis: Statistical analysis shows a significant increase in spent time near the stimulus as compared to the time spent far from the stimulus.

RESULT

A social preference test was performed, and the time was recorded successfully. Graph results present that a significant increase in spent time near the stimulus as compared to the time spent far from the stimulus.

APPLICATIONS

1. **Pharmacological testing:** Since Zebrafish are sensitive to a broad spectrum of pharmacological substances, they may be used for drug testing. The social preference test can be used to screen various medicinal products that influence social behavior in diseases such as autism spectrum disorder and social anxiety.
2. **Genetic engineering:** Through genetic engineering, researchers may investigate how certain genes influence social behavior in Zebrafish. Methods like the process of transgenesis and CRISPR/Cas9 are well-established in Zebrafish research.
3. **Developmental studies:** A significant application of the zebrafish model lies in studying the development of social behavior. Researchers can track changes in social preferences from early developmental stages to adulthood, offering valuable insights into the origins and regulatory mechanisms underlying the maturation of social behaviors over time.

ADVANTAGES

1. **Ethologically relevant:** Zebrafish are sociable animals by nature; hence the results of this test are highly pertinent to the study of social behavior. The test's utilization of natural behaviors makes its findings more ecologically sound.
2. **Genealogical and physiological similarity:** Zebrafish share numerous genetic and physiological characteristics with human beings, thereby making them a suitable model to investigate human social behavior and related diseases.
3. **High throughput screening:** Zebrafish's extremely tiny size and the elementary nature of test preparation make it suitable for high throughput screening. It works well for large-scale research and drug screening since it can test a lot of fish rapidly.
4. **Cost-effective:** It is comparatively more economical to keep Zebrafish than mammalian models. The time, as well as expenses associated with large-scale population testing and breeding, are substantially lower due to their rapid development and high fertility rates.
5. **Behavioral consistency:** Zebrafish demonstrate consistent and quantifiable social behaviors, including shoaling (group swimming), conspecific preference, and individual recognition. These behaviors provide precise and reliable insights into their social dynamics.
6. **Minimal ethical concerns:** Compared to larger vertebrates, Zebrafish generally pose fewer concerns regarding ethics when used in research, particularly when they are still larvae. This opens the possibility of more diverse experimental manipulations.
7. **Strong quantitative data:** Strong quantitative information on issues like swimming pattern shifts, remoteness from social cues, and time spent with related species may be generated from the Zebrafish social preference test. This facilitates thorough statistical analysis and reproducibility.

LIMITATIONS

1. **Context-dependent behavior:** The social preference test findings may be greatly influenced by a variety of circumstances, including tank size, shape, illumination, and other environmental conditions. Zebrafish behavior can vary greatly depending on these parameters. To achieve repeatability, rigorous standardization of the experimental setup is necessary.
2. **Stress reactions:** Zebrafish may have stress reactions that skew the findings because they are sensitive to handle. It may be difficult to discern between stress-induced behaviors and typical social preferences since stress may alter social behavior.
3. **Genetic background variability:** In Zebrafish, social behavior may be influenced by genetic background. Inconsistent outcomes may be caused by

variations both within and across Zebrafish strains, therefore careful fish selection and breeding needs to be carried out to preserve genetic consistency.

4. **Developmental stage differences:** Depending on their developmental stage, Zebrafish's social behavior might differ greatly. It might be challenging to compare social preferences across various developmental stages since larvae, juveniles, and adults may display distinct preferences.

5. **Individual variation:** Even if the Zebrafish is of the same strain and age, there may be notable individual variations in their social behavior. Due to the potential for individual variability to enhance data noise, higher sample sizes may be necessary to identify meaningful impacts.

6. **Ethical concerns:** Research on Zebrafish raises certain ethical questions, even though less queries than research on mammals. This is especially true when it comes to the possibility of stress and injury to the fish. It is essential for researchers to comply with ethical standards and guarantee the humane handling of animals.

7. **Measurement difficulties:** It may be difficult to measure social preference accurately, particularly in high-throughput settings. Although automated tracking systems are often used, they may misread motions or interactions and need to be calibrated precisely.

8. **Social preference interpretation:** Determining what specifically constitutes a "preference" can be challenging. For example, increased time spent with conspecifics may indicate social attraction, but it could also reflect anxiety or a desire for group protection. To clarify the underlying motivations, additional controls, and a rigorous experimental design are necessary.

9. **Restricted lifespan:** Zebrafish have a very limited life span which may be both a benefit and a drawback. It may also restrict long-term research on the impact of the social environment on ageing and long-term behaviour, even while it facilitates quick generational studies.

10. **Technological and resource requirements:** Specialized facilities and equipment, such as modern imaging systems and well-controlled aquatic conditions, are needed to conduct the social preference test with Zebrafish. For some research labs, this might be a hindrance.

PRACTICE QUESTIONS

1. What is called a stimulus?
2. How many fishes can sufficiently be considered for stimulus?
3. What are the ideal requirements for a social preference test tank?
4. What is a demo tank and what is a test tank?
5. What is the habituation phase?
6. What is the minimum time to habituate a fish?

REFERENCES

[1] Oliveira RF. Mind the fish: Zebrafish as a model in cognitive social neuroscience. Front Neural Circuits 2013; 7: 131.
[http://dx.doi.org/10.3389/fncir.2013.00131] [PMID: 23964204]

[2] Ogi A, Licitra R, Naef V, *et al.* Social preference tests in zebrafish: A systematic review. Front Vet Sci 2021; 7: 590057.
[http://dx.doi.org/10.3389/fvets.2020.590057] [PMID: 33553276]

[3] Dreosti E, Lopes G, Kampff AR, Wilson SW. Development of social behavior in young zebrafish. Front Neural Circuits 2015; 9: 39.
[http://dx.doi.org/10.3389/fncir.2015.00039] [PMID: 26347614]

[4] Velkey AJ, Boles J, Betts TK, Kay H, Henenlotter R, Wiens KM. High fidelity: Assessing zebrafish (*Danio rerio*) responses to social stimuli across several levels of realism. Behav Processes 2019; 164: 100-8.
[http://dx.doi.org/10.1016/j.beproc.2019.04.012] [PMID: 31022508]

[5] Velkey AJ, Koon CH, Danstrom IA, Wiens KM. Female zebrafish (*Danio rerio*) demonstrate stronger preference for established shoals over newly-formed shoals in the three-tank open-swim preference test. PLoS One 2022; 17(9): e0265703.
[http://dx.doi.org/10.1371/journal.pone.0265703] [PMID: 36129935]

[6] Pham M, Raymond J, Hester J, *et al.,* Assessing social behavior phenotypes in adult zebrafish: Shoaling, social preference, and mirror biting tests. Zebrafish protocols for neurobehavioral research. 2012: 231-46.

CHAPTER 9

Mirror Chamber Test in Zebrafish

Falguni Goel[1]**, Omkar Kumar Kuwar**[1]**, Sania Grover**[1] and **Shamsher Singh**[1,*]

[1] *Neuropharmacology Division, Department of Pharmacology, ISF College of Pharmacy, Moga, Punjab 142001, India*

INTRODUCTION

Aim: To check the anxiety-like behavior in adult Zebrafish using the mirror chamber test apparatus.

Scope and outcomes: This experiment allows us to assess anxiety-like behavior in zebrafish, particularly in response to social stimuli and novel situations. Zebrafish exhibiting anxiety-like behavior may find social interactions challenging or uncomfortable, displaying signs of anticipatory anxiety and situation avoidance. These behaviors may manifest as a reluctance to approach the mirror reduced exploration, or withdrawal from reflective areas. Such nervousness can be specific to certain social contexts or extend to encompass a broader range of interactions, providing valuable insights into the zebrafish's emotions and behavioral states under experimental conditions.

Theory: The mirror chamber test is also known as the mirror biting test. It is a well-established method for evaluating behavioral assays, such as boldness or aggressiveness, employed in the study of social behavior, self-recognition, and various neuropsychiatric and neurodevelopmental investigations in animals, including Zebrafish [1].

This apparatus typically comprises a tank with mirrored walls on one or more sides, enabling the Zebrafish to observe its reflection. The mirror chamber facilitates assessments of anxiogenic and anxiolytic effects and allows for the examination of how genetic and strain variations influence anxious behavior [2]. The mirror chamber test apparatus is shown in Fig. (**9.1**).

* **Corresponding author Shamsher Singh:** Neuropharmacology Division, Department of Pharmacology, ISF College of Pharmacy, Moga, Punjab 142001, India; Tel: +91-9779980588; E-mail: shamshersinghbajwa@gmail.com

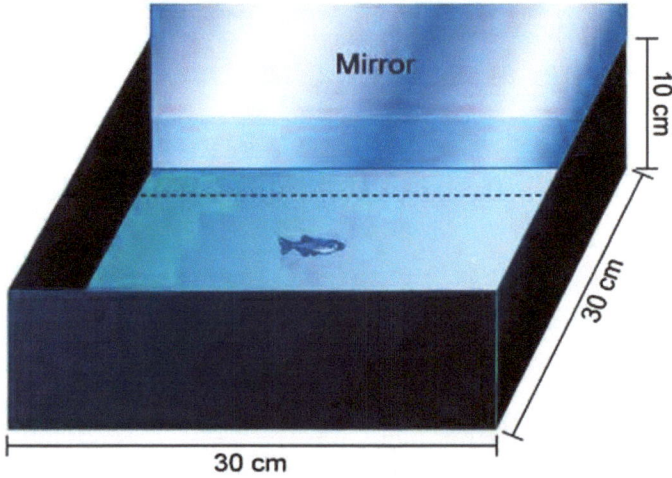

Fig. (9.1). Diagrammatic illustration of the mirror chamber.

REQUIREMENTS

Animal: Adult Zebrafish

Equipment: Mirror chamber test apparatus, ANY-maze, Camera, Graph-pad-prism.

PROCEDURE

1. Prepare the mirror chamber by rinsing it thoroughly with tap water.
2. Fill the mirror chamber with fresh water up to the designated level, ensuring that it does not exceed the capacity that will obstruct side viewing if the Zebrafish swims above the mirrored section.
3. Carefully transfer a healthy Zebrafish from the main aquarium to the mirror chamber filled with fresh water using a Fish net.
4. Ensure minimal disturbance and maintain a quiet environment throughout the experimental procedure.
5. Allow the Zebrafish to acclimate in the apparatus for 5 to 10 minutes.
6. Position the camera to record and analyze the fish's behaviour over 10 minutes.
7. Record the time spent near to the mirror or far from the mirror.
8. Behavioural indicators of anxiety and aggression include the fish approaching the mirror and attempting to attack its reflection.

Experimental setup: The Zebrafish is introduced into the mirror chamber and allowed to freely explore throughout the chamber. The fish can observe its reflection in the mirrors and interact with it as if it were another conspecific [3].

Behavioral observations: This is used to observe and record the behavior of the Zebrafish during its interaction with the mirror. Behavioral parameters such as time spent near the mirror, frequency, and duration of interactions with the reflection, and specific behaviors (*e.g.*, aggression, courtship displays) are measured. Dummy observation data are given in Table **9.1**.

Assessment of self-recognition: Self-recognition in Zebrafish is inferred based on their responses to the mirror image. If the fish demonstrates behaviors indicative of recognizing themselves, such as repeated inspection of body parts not normally visible (*e.g.*, gill covers), displaying social behaviors towards their reflection, or engaging in aggressive or courtship displays, it suggests self-awareness.

Control conditions: Control experiments may involve placing a non-reflective object (*e.g.*, a plain wall) instead of a mirror to assess whether the observed behaviors are specific to the presence of the reflective surface [3].

Experimental conditions: The mirror chamber experiment can be conducted under different experimental conditions to investigate the effects of factors such as genetic mutations, drug treatments, environmental manipulations, or social experiences on Zebrafish self-recognition and social behavior [4].

Data analysis: Data collected from the mirror chamber experiment are analyzed statistically to determine significant differences in behavior between experimental groups or conditions. This analysis can provide insights into the cognitive abilities, neural circuits, and genetic factors underlying self-awareness and social behavior in Zebrafish.

Table 9.1. Observation table of time spent near or far from the mirror on mirror chamber apparatus of Zebrafish.

S. No.	Time Spent Near the Mirror in Seconds	Time Spent Far From the Mirror in Seconds
1.	260	340
2.	230	370
3.	265	335
4.	306	294
5.	320	280
6.	220	380
7.	340	260
Mean	277.3±45.73	322.7±45.61

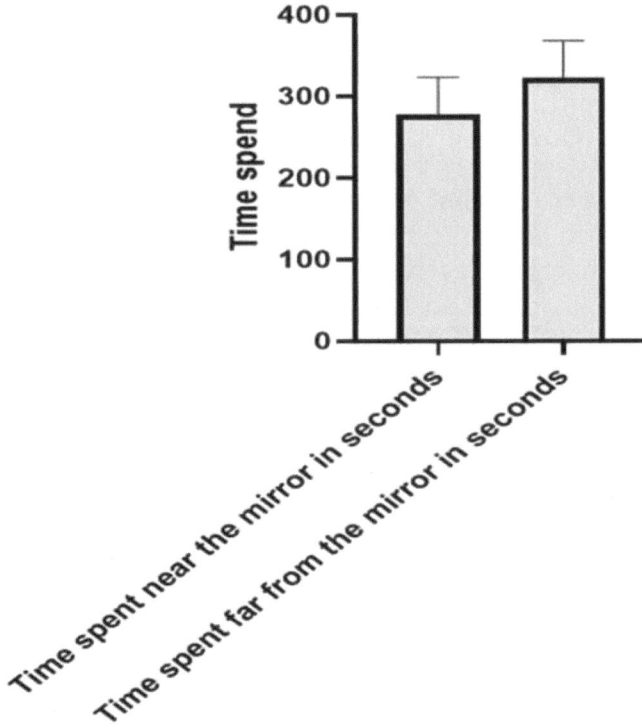

Statistical analysis: Statistical analysis shows that significantly more time is spent far from the mirror as compared to spent time near of mirror.

RESULT

A mirror chamber was performed, and the time was recorded successfully. The results indicate that the mirror chamber test effectively discriminates anxiety-like behaviors in adult zebrafish as they spent less time near the mirror as compared to time spent far from the mirror, which provides insights into the behavioral effects of this experiment.

APPLICATIONS

1. **Testing for pharmacological effects:** The mirror chamber test is sensitive to pharmacological interference and can be utilized to evaluate the effects of drugs on aggressive and social behaviours. This provides researchers with valuable insights for psychopharmacological studies [3, 4].
2. **Measurement of stress and anxiety:** The examination could reveal insights into an individual's levels of stress and the exam might provide information about a person's degree of stress and anxiety. Reduced engagement with the

mirror might signify higher stress, while an increase in avoidance or hyperactive behaviours can indicate heightened anxiety [3, 4].

3. **Research on aggressiveness:** Using the mirror chamber eliminates the ethical dilemmas and unpredictability that come with using live conspecifics in aggressiveness studies. The exam offers a regulated setting for reliably evaluating aggressive behaviour [3, 4].

ADVANTAGES

1. **Minimal instruction needed:** Zebrafish may react to their mirror without requiring a great deal of instruction. The test is easy to administer as there is a strong and quick natural reaction to a perceived conspecific.
2. **Reproducible**; The behaviours evoked in the mirror chamber, such as the length of certain behaviours (*e.g.*, circling, nipping), the frequency of assaults on the reflection, and the amount of time spent near the mirror, are readily measurable and reproducible. Measurements become objective and repeatable as a result.
3. **Controlled environment:** The test offers a controlled setting where irrelevant factors may be reduced, guaranteeing that the behaviours shown are mostly reactions to the mirror image.
4. **Speedy data collection:** The mirror chamber's behaviours are quickly seen and documented, enabling speedy data gathering and analysis. This is especially helpful when big datasets are required or when research has a tight deadline.
5. **Cost-effective:** The mirror chamber test is a cost-effective approach for behavioral research since it doesn't need specialized equipment, and Zebrafish are quite cheap to keep as compared with mice or rats.
6. **Non-invasive:** Compared to tests that require the fish to physically engage with conspecifics, the mirror chamber test is non-invasive, which lowers the possibility of harm or excessive stress for the fish.
7. **High throughput screening:** High throughput screening is made possible by the mirror chamber setup's simplicity. It is possible to test many fish at once, which makes it possible to conduct extensive research and get data quickly.

LIMITATIONS

1. **Artificial stimulus:** While not perfectly replicating the intricacy of interactions with a genuine conspecific, the mirror does offer an artificial stimulus. When confronted with their reflection, Zebrafish may not display all their typical social behaviours, which might reduce the test's ecological validity.
2. **Limited behavioral repertoire:** Compared to interactions with actual conspecifics, interactions with a mirror may only elicit specific behaviours, such as aggressiveness or curiosity, and may not well represent other social behaviours, such as mating or schooling.

3. **Interpretation ambiguity:** Reactions to a mirror image might sometimes evoke unclear behaviours. It is difficult to draw firm conclusions when there is more contact with the mirror since it might be seen as either greater hostility or heightened social interest.

4. **Stress induction:** Zebrafish may experience stress or anxiety when viewing their mirror image, particularly if they perceive the reflection as an intruder in their territory. This stress response can confound the data, making it challenging to distinguish between stress-induced activity and genuine social behavior. Zebrafish may gradually habituate to the mirror, leading to reduced responsiveness during repeated trials. This limits the test's applicability for long-term studies that require regular assessments.

5. **Individual variability:** Individual Zebrafish reactions to the mirror can vary significantly based on factors such as sex, age, and previous social experiences. These variations may introduce additional noise into the data, complicating analysis and interpretation.

6. **No real interaction feedback:** Unlike interactions with real fish, the mirror image does not provide reciprocal social signals or feedback. This lack of dynamic interaction may limit the range of observable responses and alter the natural course of social behavior.

7. **Misinterpretation potential:** Some Zebrafish may fail to recognize the mirror image as another fish and instead engage in non-social behaviours, such as exploring the mirrored surface or attempting to escape. This can lead to misinterpretation of the data, potentially affecting the validity of the results.

8. **Technical difficulties:** Setting up the mirror chamber to produce a clean, distortion-free mirror image can be challenging. Any imperfections in the setup may influence the behavior of the fish, potentially compromising the accuracy of the observations.

9. **Impact of external elements:** The behaviour of Zebrafish in the mirror chamber can be significantly influenced by external factors such as lighting, water quality, and tank configuration. Therefore, strict control and standardization of experimental conditions are essential to ensure reliable and reproducible results.

PRACTICE QUESTIONS

1. What is the use of a mirror in this test?
2. How will you measure the time spent near the mirror?
3. In which disease model mirror chamber can be used?
4. What is the habituation time for the mirror chamber?

REFERENCES

[1]   Ogi A, Licitra R, Naef V, *et al.* Social preference tests in zebrafish: A systematic review. Front Vet Sci 2021; 7: 590057.

[http://dx.doi.org/10.3389/fvets.2020.590057] [PMID: 33553276]

[2]   Way GP, Ruhl N, Snekser JL, Kiesel AL, McRobert SP. A comparison of methodologies to test aggression in zebrafish. Zebrafish 2015; 12(2): 144-51.
[http://dx.doi.org/10.1089/zeb.2014.1025] [PMID: 25621988]

[3]   Diakos E, Chevalier C, Shahjahan M, *et al.* Early impact of domestication on aggressiveness, activity, and stress behaviors in zebrafish (*Danio rerio*) using mirror test and automated videotracking. Sci Rep 2024; 14(1): 21036.
[http://dx.doi.org/10.1038/s41598-024-71451-x] [PMID: 39251766]

[4]   Axling J, Vossen LE, Peterson E, Winberg S. Boldness, activity, and aggression: Insights from a large-scale study in Baltic salmon (*Salmo salar* L). PLoS One 2023; 18(7): e0287836.
[http://dx.doi.org/10.1371/journal.pone.0287836] [PMID: 37471414]

CHAPTER 10

Three-Chamber Test in Zebrafish

Dhrita Chatterjee[1] and **Shamsher Singh**[1,*]

[1] *Neuropharmacology Division, Department of Pharmacology, ISF College of Pharmacy, Moga, Punjab 142001, India*

INTRODUCTION

Aim: To check the memory function and other behavioral activities by using a three-chambered apparatus.

Scope and outcomes: This apparatus is widely used to study memory function, spatial learning activities, depression, and anxiety-like behavior.

Theory: The three-chamber paradigm is a standard method used to assess spatial and non-spatial learning and memory in Zebrafish. This test is particularly relevant for identifying cognitive disabilities in various neurodevelopmental disorders.

It is a modified version of the T-maze apparatus, consisting of three interlinked chambers. Two side chambers are green and red from the inside with a transparent chamber present between both these 2 chambers. The apparatus has two vertical sliding windows for entering into both the left and right chambers. The size of these two slides is approximately 12× 10 cm (height × width) (Fig. **10.1**) [1].

Eddins *et al.* (2009) constructed the most updated version of the three-chambered test to examine the impact of nicotine on the cognitive abilities of the fish. It is a Plexiglas maze having a length of 44cm, height of 40 cm, width of 22 cm and it is installed inside a fish tank [2].

REQUIREMENTS

Animal: Adult Zebrafish

Equipment: Three-chambered apparatus, Any maze software, Graph pad prism, and a Camera.

---

* **Corresponding author Shamsher Singh:** Neuropharmacology Division, Department of Pharmacology, ISF College of Pharmacy, Moga, Punjab 142001, India; Tel: +91-9779980588; E-mail: shamshersinghbajwa@gmail.com

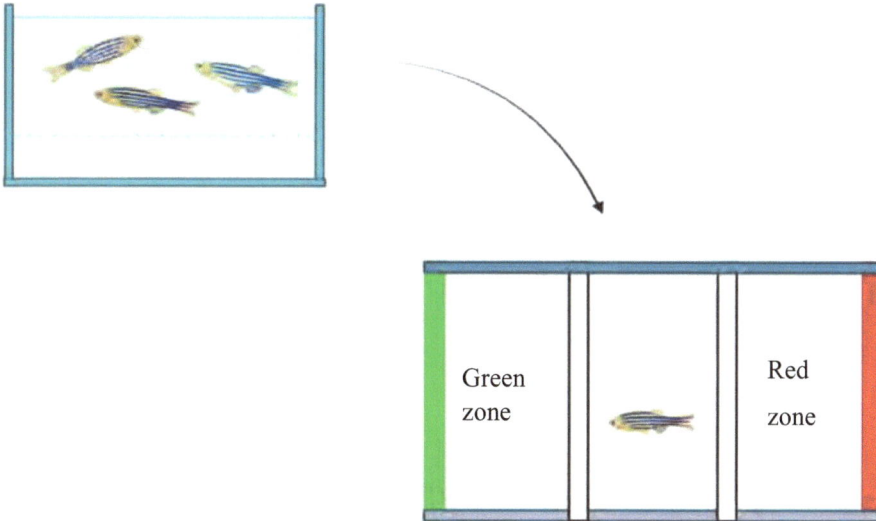

Fig. (10.1). Three-chamber test apparatus.

PROCEDURE

1. The Zebrafish is placed in the 'start zone' and allowed to freely explore the transparent chamber for 2 minutes before the test begins.
2. This phase is repeated 2-3 times to reduce experimental stress.
3. After completion of the habituation phase, Zebrafish is pushed towards the red chamber by opening the sliding door and it is allowed to remain there for at least 5 minutes.
4. In the red chamber, the fish is irritated with the help of a glass rod.
5. After 5 minutes, allow the fish to move towards the hybrid chamber without disturbances, where they remain stable in a calm and non-disturbing environment.
6. After 5 minutes, the fish is pushed to the green chamber for 5 minutes, and during this phase, it is rewarded with feed.
7. After the training phase, the fish is left to rest in the tank water for about 5 minutes.
8. In the testing phase, the fish is placed in the start zone again, and its chamber preference is recorded for 5 minutes [3].
9. Put the data on the observation table (Table **10.1**) and draw a graph by putting these data.

OBSERVATION

The observation parameter (Dummy analysis) is described in Table **10.1**.

Table 10.1. Observation table of number of entries and time of exploration on the three chamber test of Zebrafish.

Fish. No	No of Entries in the Red Zone	Time Spent in the Red Zone (Sec)	No. of Entries in the Green Zone	Time Spent in the Green Zone (Sec)
1.	5	56	7	78
2.	8	65	10	89
3.	7	62	8	92
4.	9	76	14	94
5.	8	68	16	85
Mean	7.4±1.5	65.6±7.4	11±3.8	87.6±6.3

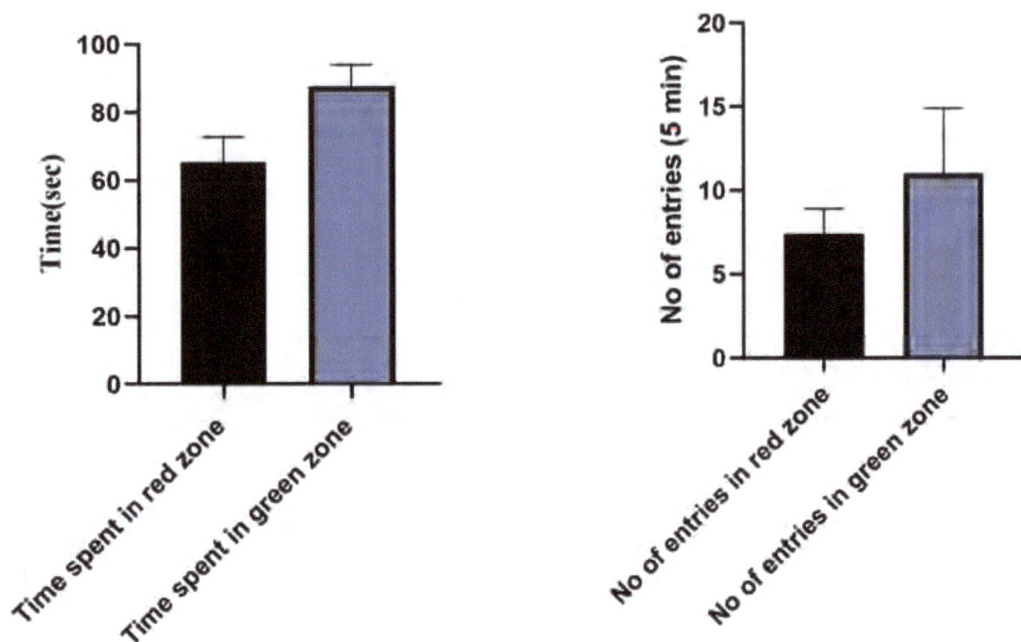

Statistical analysis: Statistical analysis indicates that both the number of entries and the time spent in the green zone have risen, while the number of entries and time spent in the red zone have decreased.

RESULT

The memory of Zebrafish using three-chamber test was performed successfully and studied carefully. The result shows that both the number of entries and the time spent in the green zone have risen, while the number of entries and time spent in the red zone have decreased.

APPLICATIONS

1. **Behavioural assessment:** The test is used to check the behaviour of fish towards color and associated stimuli.
2. **Quantitative analysis:** The instrument enables an authorized environment for analysing social activity including preference, shoaling behavior, and allowing quantitative assessment of these behaviours [3].

ADVANTAGES

1. **High efficiency:** By permitting several Zebrafish to be evaluated at the same time, the three-chamber test increases data collecting efficiency.
2. **Drug screening:** This test is performed to determine the effect of various drugs and the memory and cognition of Zebrafish.
3. **Relevance to human models:** The three-chamber test effectively evaluates social behavior, preference, and interaction, reflecting traits relevant to human social cognition.

LIMITATIONS

1. **Environmental condition:** Temperature, and noise may disturb the behaviour of the animal and may interpret the result.
2. **Physical condition of the animal:** Continuously opening and closing the sliding door may harm the animal while exploring.

PRACTICE QUESTIONS

1. What are the dimensions of the three-chamber apparatus?
2. Which parameters are evaluated using three maze apparatuses?
3. Describe the procedure of three maze apparatus.
4. Write down the main advantage of using a three-chamber apparatus instead of using any other memory testing apparatus.

REFERENCES

[1]   Rowe CJ, Crowley-Perry M, McCarthy E, Davidson TL, Connaughton VP. The three-chamber choice behavioral task using zebrafish as a model system. J Vis Exp 2021; (170): e61934.
        [PMID: 33938895]

[2]   Eddins D, Petro A, Williams P, Cerutti DT, Levin ED. Nicotine effects on learning in zebrafish: The role of dopaminergic systems. Psychopharmacology (Berl) 2009; 202(1-3): 103-9.
        [http://dx.doi.org/10.1007/s00213-008-1287-4] [PMID: 18716760]

[3]   Clevenger T, Paz J, Stafford A, Amos D, Hayes AW. An evaluation of Zebrafish, an emerging model analyzing the effects of toxicants on cognitive and neuromuscular function. Int J Toxicol 2024; 43(1): 46-62.
        [http://dx.doi.org/10.1177/10915818231207966] [PMID: 37903286]

CHAPTER 11

Light-Dark Chamber Test in Zebrafish

Falguni Goel[1], Nileshwar Kalia[1], Lav Goyal[1] and Shamsher Singh[1,*]

[1] *Neuropharmacology Division, Department of Pharmacology, ISF College of Pharmacy, Moga, Punjab 142001, India*

INTRODUCTION

Aim: The aim of this chapter is to check the anxiety in adult Zebrafish using a light-dark chamber.

Scope and outcomes: This chapter covers the entire investigation of anxiety evaluation in adult Zebrafish through the application of the light-dark chamber test. The behavioral assay uses the Zebrafish's innate preference for dark, protected areas to assess anxiety-like behaviors under carefully monitored conditions. We will examine the basic ideas that underpin the light-dark chamber test, including its construction and methods for assessing important behavioral traits that are suggestive of anxiety levels. The test protocols will be explained, with a focus on standard operating procedures to guarantee experimental rigor and study repeatability. The chapter will also cover the assay's uses in biomedical research, including how it might be used to investigate anxiety disorders and clarify neurological processes.

Theory: The light-dark chamber test is a widely used behavioral assay to evaluate anxiety-like behaviors in Zebrafish. This test leverages the Zebrafish's innate behavioral responses to light and dark stimuli, which are indicative of their anxiety levels and exploratory behavior. The principle behind this assay is the Zebrafish's preference for dark, safe areas and their tendency to explore brighter, potentially risky environments [1].

This apparatus consists of two compartments: a bright area and a dark area, connected by an opening that allows Zebrafish to move freely between them. Anxious fishes typically spend less time in bright areas and show reduced exploratory behavior characterized by fewer entries in the light zone [2]. Its non-invasive nature and high throughput capability make it an essential tool in behavioral neuroscience and psychopharmacology research, providing insights

---

* **Corresponding author Shamsher Singh:** Neuropharmacology Division, Department of Pharmacology, ISF College of Pharmacy, Moga, Punjab 142001, India; Tel: +91-9779980588; E-mail: shamshersinghbajwa@gmail.com

Shamsher Singh (Ed.)

into neurobiological mechanisms underlying anxiety disorders and aiding in the development of new therapeutic strategies [3].

EXPERIMENTAL SETUP

Zebrafish are placed individually or in groups in the chamber and allowed to explore freely. The behavior of the fish is recorded by using video tracking systems or observed directly (Fig. **11.1**).

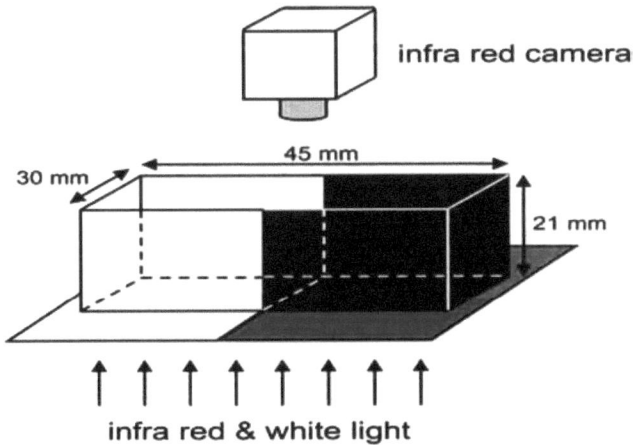

infra red camera

45 mm

30 mm

21 mm

↑ ↑ ↑ ↑ ↑ ↑ ↑ ↑
infra red & white light

Fig. (11.1). Diagram illustrating the light-dark chamber.

Assessment of light preference: Researchers analyze the amount of time Zebrafish spend in the light compartment compared to the dark compartment. An increased preference for one compartment over the other indicates a preference for that light condition.

Water quality: To prevent any confusing stimuli, make sure the water is consistently clean.

Water Temperature: Fill the maze with either tank water or a combination of tank water and filtered tap water that has been treated with conditioner up to a height of around 8 to 10 cm. The ideal water temperature range is between 25.5 and 28.5 °C, and a 25-watt heater is placed on the maze's floor to maintain temperature. It is advisable to time trials using a stopwatch. Food should be placed into the proper goal zone using stainless steel tweezers if the study involves rewards.

Behavioral parameters: Various behavioral parameters can be measured during the experiment, including:

1. Time spent in each compartment.
2. Number of transitions between compartments.
3. Swimming activity (speed, distance traveled) in each compartment.
4. Social interactions between fish in the chamber.

Experimental conditions: The light-dark chamber experiment can be conducted under different lighting conditions (*e.g.*, different light intensity and wavelength) to study the effects of light on Zebrafish behavior. Additionally, the chamber can be used to assess the influence of factors such as genetic mutations, drug treatments, or environmental manipulations on light preference.

REQUIREMENTS

Animal: Adult Zebrafish

Equipment: Light-dark chamber apparatus, Any-maze software, Graph-pad-prism, Camera.

PROCEDURE

1. Maintain consistent environmental conditions in the experimental room, including temperature ($28 - 30$ ^{0}C), light cycle, and water quality parameters for the Zebrafish.
2. Acclimate adult Zebrafish to the experimental room for at least 30 minutes before testing to minimize stress.
3. Position the light-dark chamber in a quiet area with minimal disturbances to ensure an accurate behavioral response.
4. Carefully transfer a single adult Zebrafish from its home tank to the light-dark chamber using a net.
5. Start the timer and allow the Zebrafish to explore freely for a pre-determined duration (5 minutes). Record the session with video equipment to capture detailed behavioral responses.
6. Observe and record the behaviors, such as latency to the dark compartment and time spent in each compartment.
7. Use appropriate statistical tests to compare results between experimental groups if different test conditions are applied.

Data analysis: Data collected from the experiment can be analyzed statistically to determine significant differences in behavior between the light and dark compartments, as well as the effects of experimental variables on Zebrafish behavior.

OBSERVATION

A dummy analysis is given in Table **11.1**.

Table 11.1. Observation table of time spent in dark and light zones and latency time on the light-dark chamber apparatus of Zebrafish.

S. No.	Time Spent in the Dark Zone n Seconds	Time Spent in the Light Zone in Seconds	Latency Time to First Crossing in Seconds
1.	150	50	20
2.	180	30	15
3.	120	80	25
4.	140	60	18
5.	160	40	22
6.	135	65	19
Mean	150.7±20.90	52.86±16.80	19.83±3.43

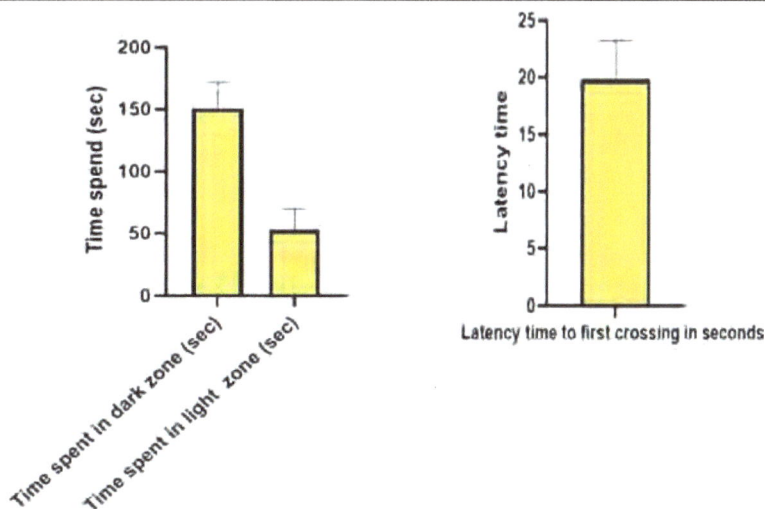

Statistical significance: Statistical analysis shows a significant increase in time spent in the dark zone as compared to the light zone.

RESULT

The results of this experiment indicate that Zebrafish show a strong preference for dark environments over light ones, which is consistent with typical anxiety responses in animal models. This behavior suggests that the light-dark chamber test can effectively be used to assess anxiety in Zebrafish.

APPLICATIONS

1. **Assessment of anxiety-like behavior:** The primary use of the light-dark chamber test is to assess the anxiety-like behaviors in Zebrafish [4]. By measuring their preference for dark, enclosed spaces over brightly lit areas, researchers can quantify anxiety-related responses such as avoidance behavior and reduced exploration in potentially anxiogenic environments.
2. **Screening for neurotoxicity:** The light-dark chamber test can serve as a tool for assessing the neurotoxic effects of chemicals or environmental pollutants [5]. Exposure to neurotoxic substances may induce changes in anxiety-related behaviors in Zebrafish, providing insights into potential hazards to neurological health.
3. **Pharmacological screening:** The test is valuable for screening and evaluating the effects of pharmacological agents on anxiety-like behaviors [6]. Researchers can administer anxiolytic or anxiogenic drugs to Zebrafish and observe changes in behavior, such as alterations in the time spent in the dark compartment. This helps in identifying potential therapeutic compounds for anxiety disorders.

ADVANTAGES

1. **Measurement of anxiety:** Zebrafish typically prefer darker settings, and their behavior in the light-dark chamber mirrors anxiety levels, making it a useful way to measure anxiety-related behaviors.
2. **Fast and easy:** The test requires no preparation or handling, making it simple to perform and less stressful for the animals.
3. **Measurable data:** Enables objective analysis by providing precise, measurable data, such as the amount of time spent in each chamber, the time it takes to move between chambers, and the delay it takes to reach the dark region.
4. **High throughput:** The simple setup makes it possible to test many fish at once, which makes it appropriate for high throughput screening, particularly in pharmaceutical research.
5. **Non-intrusive:** Unlike more intrusive treatments, this test does not cause bodily injury and causes less stress.
6. **Cost-effective:** This method is affordable and only requires minimal equipment, making it suitable for a wide range of labs.
7. **Behavioral consistency:** The data is more dependable when Zebrafish react consistently and dependably in the light-dark room.
8. **Research on development and genetics:** Beneficial for examining how genetic alterations and developmental shifts affect behaviors associated with anxiety.

LIMITATIONS

1. **Restricted scope:** The Zebrafish's predilection for gloomy settings serves as the primary basis for measuring anxiety-related behaviors in this test. However, it may not provide comprehensive insights into anxiety or other behavioral factors unrelated to light-dark preference.

2. **Interpretation challenges:** Although spending longer time in the darkroom is often associated with anxiety-like behavior, other variables, such as an individual's inclination for exploration or light sensitivity, may also play a role in this behavior. This may make it more difficult to interpret the findings.

3. **Stress response:** The sudden change from bright to dark surroundings may cause stress, potentially affecting how anxiety is measured. Distinguishing between natural anxiety and stress-induced behavior may be difficult.

4. **Environmental variables:** Several environmental variables, including the size of the chambers, the water quality, and the color and intensity of the light, may affect how Zebrafish behave in the light-dark room. To ensure repeatability, these conditions must be strictly standardized.

5. **Individual variation:** Age, sex, and prior experiences may all have a substantial impact on an individual Zebrafish's reaction to the light-dark chamber. This fluctuation might exacerbate noise in the data and make statistical analysis more difficult.

6. **Genetic background:** The behavior of Zebrafish strains in the light-dark test may be influenced by genetic variations. To guarantee consistent outcomes, this calls for thorough selection and genetic background management.

7. **Restricted behavioral repertoire:** Zebrafish may display a wider variety of anxiety-related behaviors than what is possible to see in the light-dark chamber test. It might take several tests to get a more complete behavioral profile.

8. **Behavioral overlap:** It might be difficult to distinguish between certain anxiety-related behaviors when there is behavioral overlap between behaviors shown in the light-dark chamber and those seen in other tests.

PRACTICE QUESTIONS

1. What is the rationale for performing a light-dark chamber?
2. What is the measurement of light dark chamber?
3. What does the dark color represent?
4. What does the light color represent?
5. What is called latency time?

REFERENCES

[1]   Mezzomo NJ, Silveira A, Giuliani GS, Quadros VA, Rosemberg DB. The role of taurine on anxiety-like behaviors in zebrafish: A comparative study using the novel tank and the light–dark tasks. Neurosci Lett 2016; 613: 19-24.

[http://dx.doi.org/10.1016/j.neulet.2015.12.037] [PMID: 26724225]

[2]   Blaser RE, Peñalosa YM. Stimuli affecting zebrafish (*Danio rerio*) behavior in the light/dark preference test. Physiol Behav 2011; 104(5): 831-7.
[http://dx.doi.org/10.1016/j.physbeh.2011.07.029] [PMID: 21839758]

[3]   Mrinalini R, Tamilanban T, Naveen Kumar V, Manasa K. Zebrafish–the Neurobehavioural model in trend. Neuroscience 2023; 520: 95-118.
[http://dx.doi.org/10.1016/j.neuroscience.2022.12.016] [PMID: 36549602]

[4]   Maximino C, de Brito TM, da Silva Batista AW, Herculano AM, Morato S, Gouveia A Jr. Measuring anxiety in zebrafish: A critical review. Behav Brain Res 2010; 214(2): 157-71.
[http://dx.doi.org/10.1016/j.bbr.2010.05.031] [PMID: 20510300]

[5]   Quevedo C, Behl M, Ryan K, *et al.* Detection and prioritization of developmentally neurotoxic and/or neurotoxic compounds using zebrafish. Toxicol Sci 2019; 168(1): 225-40.
[http://dx.doi.org/10.1093/toxsci/kfy291] [PMID: 30521027]

[6]   Peng X, Lin J, Zhu Y, *et al.* Anxiety-related behavioral responses of pentylenetetrazole-treated zebrafish larvae to light-dark transitions 2016.
[http://dx.doi.org/10.1016/j.pbb.2016.03.010]

CHAPTER 12

Plus-Maze Test in Zebrafish

Vaishali[1], Kousik Maparu[1] and Shamsher Singh[1,*]

[1] *Neuropharmacology Division, Department of Pharmacology, ISF College of Pharmacy, Moga, Punjab 142001, India*

INTRODUCTION

Aim: The aim of this chapter is to check the anxiety-like behavior in adult Zebrafish using a plus-maze apparatus.

Scope and outcomes: This experiment provides insights into anxiety-like behavior in Zebrafish. Individuals may find extremely uncomfortable social interactions with anticipatory anxiety and a tendency to avoid certain situations. The nervousness may be restricted to certain social contexts or broadened to include nearly all social interactions.

Theory: The "+" shaped device is made up of arms with varying depths, each corresponding to varying degrees of aversiveness, similar to the elevated plus-maze [1]. The plus maze is an enclosed environment created to observe Zebrafish as they make decisions and exhibit anxiety-like behaviors [2].

This experimental configuration consists of a cross-shaped labyrinth with two enclosed and two open arms (Fig. **12.1**), allowing researchers to evaluate how Zebrafish explore and navigate the place [3].

CONDITIONS OF THE ENVIRONMENT

Lighting: To simulate open *vs.* protected environments, the closed arms should be either entirely dark or somewhat dimmed, while the open arms should be often brilliantly illuminated.

Water quality: To prevent any confusing stimuli, make sure the water remains consistently clean.

---

* **Corresponding author Shamsher Singh:** Neuropharmacology Division, Department of Pharmacology, ISF College of Pharmacy, Moga, Punjab 142001, India; Tel: +91-9779980588; E-mail: shamshersinghbajwa@gmail.com

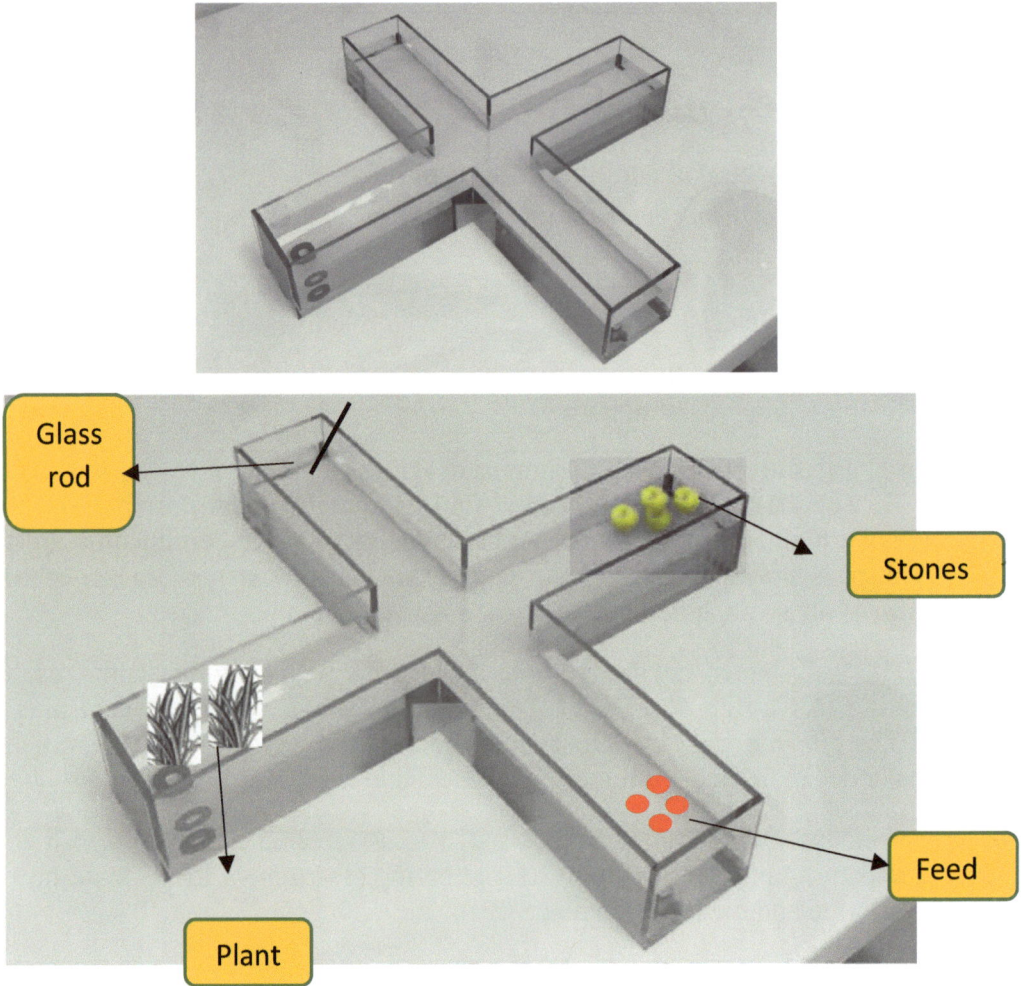

Fig. (12.1). Diagram illustrating the elevated plus maze.

Evaluation Criteria

1. **Anxiety level:** Compare the amount of time Zebrafish spend in the closed and open arms. Spending more time in the open arms indicates lesser anxiety, whereas spending more time in the closed arms is usually regarded as more anxiety level.

2. **Number of entries for every arm:** Count how many times Zebrafish enter each arm type. Increased entries in the open arms may suggest lower anxiety levels.

3. **Time to first entry:** After placing the fish in the maze, record how long it took the fish to reach the first open arm. A longer delay in entering the open arm may indicate an increased level of anxiousness.

4. **The total distance covered:** Track the total traveling distance of Zebrafish throughout the test. This may reveal anxiety-related behaviors and provide insights into overall activity levels.

5. **Investigative Behaviour:** Observe any exploratory actions, such as a Zebrafish dipping its head slightly into the open arms. These kinds of actions may provide more details regarding anxiety levels.

6. **Thigmotaxis or hugging the wall:** Record the Zebrafish's propensity to remain near the arm walls, especially while the arms are open. Elevated thigmotaxis levels are often linked to heightened anxiety.

7. **Changes in behavior:** Examine the frequency and pattern of behavioral changes between the arms. This helps in determining how exploratory behavior and anxiety-driven avoidance coexist.

8. **Freezing action:** Extended periods for freezing or immobility, particularly with arms extended, may be a sign of elevated stress or worry.

9. **Speed:** Calculate how quickly the Zebrafish go through the labyrinth. A slower gait with the fins outstretched may indicate nervousness.

10. **Risk assessment behavior:** Actions like stopping at the entrance of the open arm and looking around before going inside are examples of this behavior. Cautious behavior may indicate anxiety.

REQUIREMENTS

Animal: Adult Zebrafish

Equipment: T-maze, ANY-maze, Camera, Graph-pad-prism.

PROCEDURE

The plus maze test apparatus has three sessions: The habituation phase, the training phase, and the testing phase [4].

1. Firstly, separate one healthy Zebrafish for the procedure and remove it from the water tank.

2. Transfer the fish to the plus-maze with the help of a net.

3. Ensure that the procedure is carried out in noise noise-free environment to reduce experimental stress.

4. Allow the individual fish to habituate in the apparatus for 10 mins.

5. Now, set up the camera to record the video and analyze it for 10 minutes.

6. To create mild irritation, put a glass rod in one arm and 5-6 stones in the second arm.

7. Place food as a reward in the third arm, and in the fourth arm, insert some plants.

8. A greater number of entries of fish toward the fourth arm indicates the healthy

nature of fish.
9. In the testing phase, observe the effect of the drug on the learning and memory functioning of the fish.

Data analysis: Data collected from the plus chamber experiment are analyzed statistically to determine significant differences in behavior between experimental groups or conditions. This analysis can provide insights into the cognitive abilities, neural circuits, and genetic factors underlying self-awareness and social behavior in Zebrafish.

OBSERVATION

A dummy analysis is given in Table **12.1**.

Table 12.1. Observation table of time spent in different arms on the plus-maze apparatus of Zebrafish.

S. No.	Time Spent in I Arm (Sec)	Time Spent in II Arm (Sec)	Time Spent in III Arm (Sec)	Time Spent in Arm Iv (Sec)
01.	30	25	120	75
02.	37	22	145	90
03	31	29	180	59
04	26	34	140	84
05	33	27	91	111
Mean	31.40±4.03	27.40±4.50	135.2±32.83	83.80±19.18

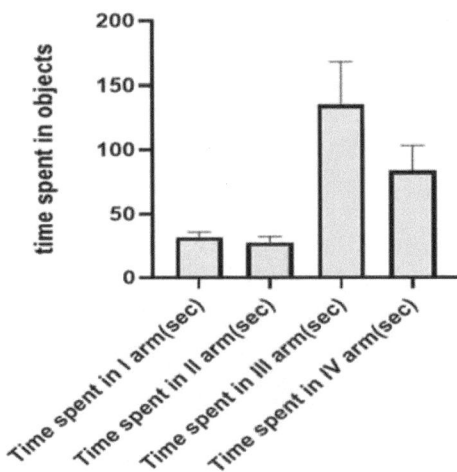

Statistical evaluation: Statistical analysis shows that the time spent in arm I and II is less compared time spent in arm III and arm IV.

RESULT

The plus maze apparatus was successfully conducted using adult Zebrafish, with careful analysis of the results. The data, as presented in the observation table, were compared based on the time spent in arm I, arm II, arm III, and arm IV. The graph demonstrates a significant increase in the time spent in arms III and IV compared to I and II.

APPLICATIONS

1. **Applications in pharmacology:** Because the plus maze test is responsive to pharmacological treatments, researchers may evaluate how different medicines affect behaviors associated with anxiety. This is especially helpful for vetting substances that may be anxiogenic or anxiolytic [5].
2. **Developmental and genetic studies:** Because Zebrafish are genetically manipulable, it is possible to examine how genetic changes affect anxiety and exploratory behavior using the plus maze test. Because Zebrafish mature quickly and allow researchers to examine changes across many life stages, it is especially helpful for developmental investigations.
3. **Behavioral consistency:** In the plus maze, Zebrafish consistently and reliably respond, which improves the validity and dependability of the data gathered.
4. **Environmental control:** Researchers can systematically adjust and examine the impact of several environmental elements, such as light intensity, color, and tank arrangement, on behavior thanks to the plus maze's controlled environment.

ADVANTAGES

1. **Quantifiable data:** The exam offers precise, objective measurements, including the amount of time spent in each arm, the number of entries, and the delay to access certain regions. This makes it possible to monitor anxiety and exploratory behaviors precisely and consistently.
2. **Non-invasive:** The test causes the least amount of stress and injury to the Zebrafish since it does not involve any major handling or surgical procedures.
3. **High throughput:** Fish may be tested simultaneously because of the plus maze setup's efficiency and simplicity. Because of this, it may be used for high-throughput screening, which is very helpful for genetic and pharmacological research.
4. **Cost-effective:** Zebrafish need little upkeep, and many labs may easily create and operate the plus maze apparatus because of its simplicity and affordability.

5. **Relevance to mammalian models:** Zebrafish share conserved neurotransmitter systems (*e.g.*, dopamine, serotonin) with mammals, but their simpler brain structure offers more accessible analysis of neural circuits.

6. **Versatility:** Besides anxiety, a broad variety of behaviors, including exploration, novelty seeking, and risk assessment, may be studied using the plus maze. It is a widely valuable tool in behavioral neuroscience because of its adaptability.

7. **Fast data collection:** The test makes it possible to gather and analyze behavioral data quickly, which makes it possible to get findings quickly and, if necessary, make fast changes to the experimental design.

LIMITATIONS

1. **Environmental sensitivity:** Several environmental elements, including illumination, water quality, and tank configuration, may have an impact on Zebrafish behavior in the plus maze. Strict standardization is necessary for this sensitivity to guarantee consistency and repeatability in the outcomes.

2. **Stress induction:** If the lighting is excessively bright or there are quick changes between open and closed arms, the test setting itself may cause stress. The perception of behaviors associated with worry may get confused by this stress.

3. **Synthetic environment:** The plus maze is a synthetic setting that could not accurately reflect the natural circumstances that Zebrafish encounter in the wild. This may reduce the results' ecological validity and their suitability for natural behaviors.

4. **Limited scope of behavior:** Arm preference and exploratory activity are the main ways in which the test assesses anxiety-related behaviors. It may not fully capture the complexities of anxiety or other associated behaviors, requiring the use of other tests to get a thorough evaluation.

5. **Individual variation:** Age, sex, and past experiences are some of the variables that might cause notable individual variations in Zebrafish's reactions to the plus maze. This fluctuation might contaminate the data with noise and make statistical analysis more difficult.

6. **Difficulties with interpretation:** Although the duration of time spent in open arms as opposed to closed arms is often considered a sign of anxiety, other variables like curiosity, sensitivity to light, or overall activity levels may also have an impact on this behavior. This may make it more difficult to understand the findings.

7. **Limited behavioral repertoire**: In contrast to more intricate social or environmental interactions, the behaviors shown in the plus maze may be more restricted, perhaps omitting significant facets of Zebrafish behavior.

8. **Potential for misinterpretation:** Some of the behaviors shown in the plus

maze, including freezing or moving less, might be mistakenly identified as signs of anxiety when they are caused by other conditions like exhaustion or ill health.

PRACTICE QUESTIONS

1. What are the different methods to irritate the fish?
2. What is the rationale for making four arms in it?
3. Why should one become socially interactive?
4. Name some anti-anxiety drugs.
5. Define anxiety.

REFERENCES

[1]   Varga ZK, Zsigmond Á, Pejtsik D, *et al.* The swimming plus-maze test: A novel high-throughput model for assessment of anxiety-related behaviour in larval and juvenile zebrafish (*Danio rerio*). Sci Rep 2018; 8(1): 16590.
       [http://dx.doi.org/10.1038/s41598-018-34989-1] [PMID: 30410116]

[2]   Walsh-Monteiro A, Pessoa RS, Sanches ÉM, *et al.* A new anxiety test for zebrafish: Plus maze with ramp. Psychol Neurosci 2016; 9(4): 457-64.
       [http://dx.doi.org/10.1037/pne0000067]

[3]   Walf AA, Frye CA. The use of the elevated plus maze as an assay of anxiety-related behavior in rodents. Nat Protoc 2007; 2(2): 322-8.
       [http://dx.doi.org/10.1038/nprot.2007.44] [PMID: 17406592]

[4]   Sison M, Gerlai R. Associative learning in zebrafish (*Danio rerio*) in the plus maze. Behav Brain Res 2010; 207(1): 99-104.
       [http://dx.doi.org/10.1016/j.bbr.2009.09.043] [PMID: 19800919]

[5]   Benvenutti R, Marcon M, Gallas-Lopes M, de Mello AJ, Herrmann AP, Piato A. Swimming in the maze: An overview of maze apparatuses and protocols to assess zebrafish behavior. Neurosci Biobehav Rev 2021; 127: 761-78.
       [http://dx.doi.org/10.1016/j.neubiorev.2021.05.027] [PMID: 34087275]

CHAPTER 13

Y-Maze Test in Zebrafish

Dhrita Chatterjee[1], Kousik Maparu[1] and Shamsher Singh[1,*]

[1] Neuropharmacology Division, Department of Pharmacology, ISF College of Pharmacy, Moga, Punjab 142001, India

INTRODUCTION

Aim: The aim of this chapter is to investigate the memory and cognition of adult Zebrafish using the Y maze apparatus.

Scope and outcome: This practical technique allows us to assess spatial memory by examining cognitive and behavioral parameters, such as the tendency of a fish to explore novel places. By performing the test, researchers can investigate the behavior of fish, such as environmental stimuli, exploration tendencies, spatial memory, and decision-making capabilities. The outcomes of the Y maze test can improve our knowledge in the fields of biology, neurology, and drug discovery.

Theory: The Zebrafish 'Y' maze apparatus is considered an aquatic adaptation of the traditional Y maze used for rodents. It is in the shape of capital 'Y' and used for evaluating the spatial working memory by analyzing the behavior of the fish during the procedure. This setup was first confirmed to be genuine in research conducted by Cognato *et al.* (2012).

The aquatic Y-shaped tank is made up of glass or acrylic materials with three arms of equal length. The length of each arm is 25 cm, width 8 cm, height 15 cm, and having a 120° angle between them (Fig. **13.1**). Compared to the T maze (where the arms have a 90° angle), it provides more area for fluid movement and exploration, which reduces the learning time. To accomplish the goal, food is used as a reward, and animals are forced to follow a particular search pattern or reduce the time or error while seeking the reward.

***** **Corresponding author Shamsher Singh:** Neuropharmacology Division, Department of Pharmacology, ISF College of Pharmacy, Moga, Punjab 142001, India; Tel: +91-9779980588; E-mail: shamshersinghbajwa@gmail.com

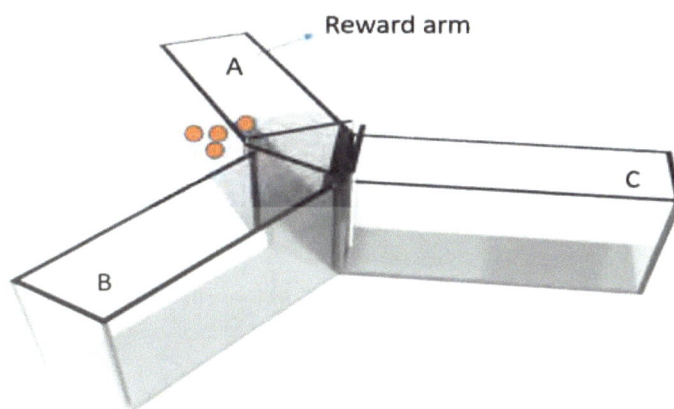

Fig. (13.1). Y-Maze test apparatus.

Each fish is placed at the starting point of the maze and allowed to explore. The three arms are equipped with doors at the entrance of each arm, which prevents the fish from entering more than one arm. If the fish reaches the reward zone in the first trial, then it is expected to explore another zone in the next trial. The capability of choosing the alternate arm determines the decision-making capabilities of the fish and the location-specific memory. The number of arm entries and the time the Zebrafish stays in each arm are recorded [1].

REQUIREMENTS

Animal: Adult Zebrafish

Equipment: Y-maze, ANY-maze, Camera, Graph-pad-prism.

PROCEDURE

1. Before beginning the test, set up the Y maze apparatus in a noise-free environment and fill the maze with system water from their home tank.
2. Before testing, habituate the fish to the maze by allowing it to freely explore throughout the maze to minimize experimental stress.
3. Observe the behavior of the animal and record which arm it mainly prefers.
4. Begin the pre-training phase, where the animal is introduced into the apparatus with a food reward in one of the arms.
5. The animal chooses the reward arm in the first trial. Then, in the second trial, the previous reward arm is closed, and then the animal is introduced to the apparatus and allowed to explore the end of the arm.

6. Food is placed in the alternative arm during the second trial. Repeat this process for an equal amount of time. This pre-training phase continues for about 3 minutes.
7. Then, in the testing phase, food is placed in both arms, and all three doors are open.
8. Observe the choice of the fish. If the fish chooses arm A, which means the correct arm choice, then it is rewarded with food.
9. And if it chooses arm B, then it will receive no reward. Thus, the decision-making capability of fish is determined.
10. If the fish does not choose any arm between A and B and stays in arm C, it means no decision-making capability of the fish is determined.
11. All the procedure is recorded to observe the behaviour of the animal. Collect data on different parameters like the number of entries to each arm and the time spent in arm A as well as arm B.
12. Ensure that all the procedures follow ethical guidelines to minimize the experimental stress of the animal [2].

Data Analysis

1. Review the previously recorded video and determine the type of behavioral nature shown by the fish during the experiment.
2. All study videos are recorded and analyzed in a spreadsheet.
3. Perform statistical evaluation to compare the obtained data about spending time in the A-arm (reward zone) and the B-arm (not reward zone).
4. Data should be checked by two independent study coordinators to keep the study from bias and produce more scientific as well as relevant data from the experiment.

CONDITIONS OF THE ENVIRONMENT

Water Quality: Ensure the water is kept clean to avoid any potential confounding stimuli.

Water Temperature: Fill the maze with either tank water or a combination of tank water and filtered tap water that has been treated with conditioner up to a height of around 8 to 10 cm. The ideal water temperature range is between 25.5 and 28.5 °C, and a 25-watt heater is placed on the maze's floor to maintain temperature. It is advisable to time trials using a stopwatch. Food should be placed into the proper goal zone using stainless steel tweezers if the study involves rewards [3].

OBSERVATION

A dummy analysis is given in Table **13.1**.

Table 13.1. Observation table of the time spent in Arms A, B, and C and the number of times the line is crossed on the Y-maze apparatus by Zebrafish.

S. No.	Time Spent in Each Arm (Sec.)			No. of Times the Line is Crossed
	Arm A	Arm B	Arm C	
`1.	6	5	8	2
2.	8	8	9	2
3.	7	6	8	2
4.	9	7	7	2
5.	6	7	5	2
Mean	7.2±1.3	6.6±1.1	7.4±1.5	2.0±0.0

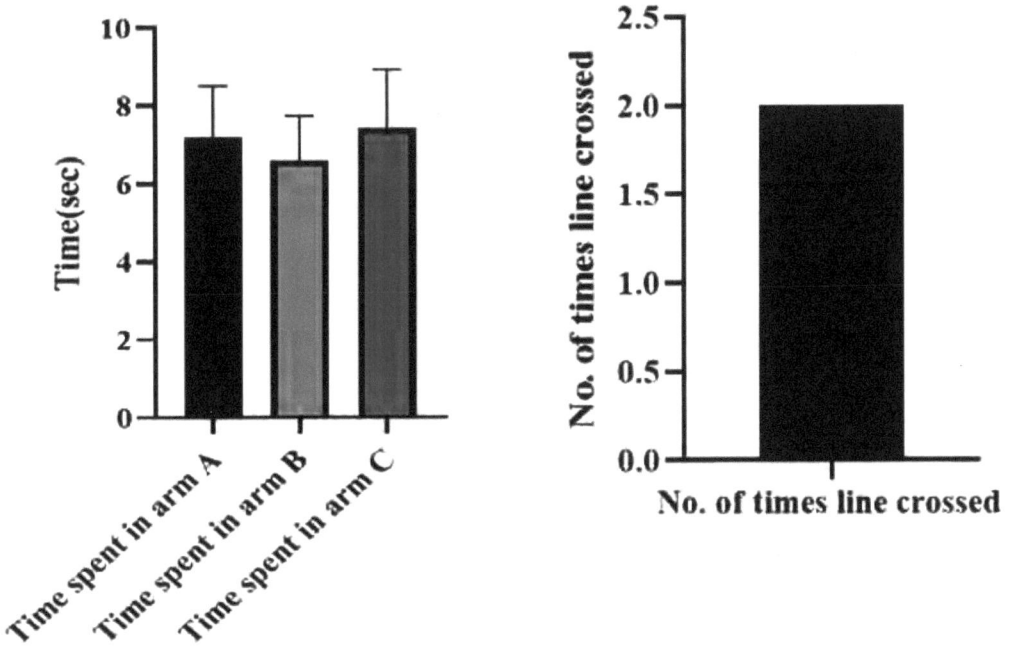

Statistical analysis: Statistical analysis shows that the time spent in arm A is more compared to arm B and arm C.

RESULT

The Y maze apparatus was successfully conducted using adult Zebrafish, with careful analysis of the results. The data, as presented in the observation table, were compared based on the time spent in arm A, arm B, and arm C. The graph demonstrates a significant increase in the time spent in arm A compared to B and C.

APPLICATIONS

1. **Studying neurodegenerative diseases:** Neurodegenerative disorders, including Parkinson's and Alzheimer's, are modeled in Zebrafish, and their effects on cognitive function are evaluated through learning tests.
2. **Pharmacological screening:** Learning tests are used to identify neurotoxic and neuroprotective substances that affect Zebrafish memory and learning.
3. **Genetic manipulation:** Learning tests are used to investigate the genetic basis of memory and learning in Zebrafish, which are genetically manipulable.
4. **Behavioral neuroscience:** Behavioral neuroscience, including anxiety-like behavior and locomotor activity in Zebrafish, is studied using learning tests.
5. **Cognitive research:** Cognitive functions like associative learning, object recognition, and spatial recognition are studied in Zebrafish.
6. **High-throughput screening:** In high-throughput screening, learning tests are employed to find novel chemicals that impact Zebrafish memory and learning [4].

ADVANTAGES

1. **Less learning time:** The Y maze apparatus is simpler compared to the T maze; it reduces the learning time.
2. **Simple setup:** The Y maze is simple and economical to set up, providing more space for exploration throughout the apparatus.
3. **Behavioral assessment:** By performing the test, multiple behavioral parameters are examined, including spatial memory, cognition, and decision-making capabilities.
4. **Non-invasive:** As this procedure requires less training, it is considered a non-invasive technique among all behavioral parameters.
5. **Productive learning:** Learning efficiency is faster in the Y maze as compared to the T maze because the Y maze has a 120° angle between two arms while the T maze has a 90° angle.
6. **Less training period:** This test requires a less training period in comparison with other behavioral parameters.
7. **Natural Preference:** As the Y maze is the simpler version of the T maze, animals are explored throughout the maze based on their innate behavior.

8. **Genetic and Pharmacological-related Research:** This test investigates the impact of drugs or genetic mutations on Zebrafish behavior, drawing parallels to similar effects observed in mammals.

LIMITATIONS

1. **Environmental condition:** Environmental conditions such as noise and temperature can affect the result of the test.
2. **High chance of error:** This test exhibits a high chance of error.
3. **Increased Stress:** Sometimes, the procedure of the Y maze apparatus may increase the experimental stress in fish.
4. **Handling and training:** Improper handling of fish during the experiment may interpret the result of the experiment.
5. **Limited to short-term memory:** Using the Y maze apparatus, only short-term memory is evaluated. It may not be relevant for assessing long-term memory [5].

PRACTICE QUESTIONS

1. What are the ideal dimensions of the apparatus used for the Y-maze test in Zebrafish?
2. What are the advantages of performing the Y-maze test in Zebrafish?
3. What are the 3 phases involved in performing the Y-maze test in fish?
4. In the Y-maze test, which parts of the brain are potentially involved?
5. Describe in brief the procedure of the Y-maze in fish.
6. What are the possible applications of the Y-maze test in fish?

REFERENCES

[1]   Cognato GP, Bortolotto JW, Blazina AR, *et al.* Y-Maze memory task in zebrafish (*Danio rerio*): The role of glutamatergic and cholinergic systems on the acquisition and consolidation periods. Neurobiol Learn Mem 2012; 98(4): 321-8.
        [http://dx.doi.org/10.1016/j.nlm.2012.09.008] [PMID: 23044456]

[2]   Benvenutti R, Marcon M, Gallas-Lopes M, de Mello AJ, Herrmann AP, Piato A. Swimming in the maze: An overview of maze apparatuses and protocols to assess zebrafish behavior. Neurosci Biobehav Rev 2021; 127: 761-78.
        [http://dx.doi.org/10.1016/j.neubiorev.2021.05.027] [PMID: 34087275]

[3]   Aoki R, Tsuboi T, Okamoto H. Y-maze avoidance: An automated and rapid associative learning paradigm in zebrafish. Neurosci Res 2015; 91: 69-72.
        [http://dx.doi.org/10.1016/j.neures.2014.10.012] [PMID: 25449146]

[4]   Kraeuter AK, Guest PC, Sarnyai Z. The Y-maze for assessment of spatial working and reference memory in mice. Pre-clinical models: Techniques and protocols. 2019: 105-11.

[5]   Cleal M, Fontana BD, Ranson DC, *et al.* The Free-movement pattern Y-maze: A cross-species measure of working memory and executive function. Behav Res Methods 2021; 53(2): 536-57.
        [http://dx.doi.org/10.3758/s13428-020-01452-x] [PMID: 32748238]

CHAPTER 14

Square-Maze Test in Zebrafish

Falguni Goel[1], Lovekesh Singh[1] and Shamsher Singh[1,*]

[1] *Neuropharmacology Division, Department of Pharmacology, ISF College of Pharmacy, Moga, Punjab 142001, India*

INTRODUCTION

Aim: The aim of this chapter is to check the anxiety-like behavior in adult Zebrafish by using a square maze test apparatus.

Scope and outcomes: This practical will allow us to investigate anxiety-like behavior in Zebrafish. The square maze is a widely used behavioral assay for *Danio rerio*, employed to study various aspects of behavior, including anxiety, exploration, learning, and memory.

Theory: The Square Cognitive Maze (SCM) is a tool used to assess cognitive abilities in animals, including Zebrafish [1]. It consists of a square tank divided into four equal-sized sections, each containing 12 centimeters of water maintained at a temperature of 37°C (Fig. **14.1**). Food incentives are placed in the fourth section to motivate the fish to learn the location of the reward [2].

EXPERIMENTAL CONSIDERATIONS

1. **Consistent lighting and environment:** Ensure consistent environmental conditions to minimize variability in behavior due to external factors.
2. **Acclimation period:** Allow Zebrafish to acclimate to the maze environment before starting measures to reduce stress-induced behavior changes.
3. **Control groups:** Use control groups to compare against experimental groups, ensuring that observed behaviors are due to the experimental manipulation and no other variables.

CONDITIONS OF THE ENVIRONMENT

Water Quality: To prevent any confusing stimuli, make sure the water is consistently clean.

---

* **Corresponding author Shamsher Singh:** Neuropharmacology Division, Department of Pharmacology, ISF College of Pharmacy, Moga, Punjab 142001, India; Tel: +91-9779980588; E-mail: shamshersinghbajwa@gmail.com

Water Temperature: Fill the maze with either tank water or a combination of tank water and filtered tap water that has been treated with conditioner up to a height of around 8 to 10 cm. The ideal water temperature range is between 25.5 and 28.5 °C, and a 25-watt heater is placed on the maze's floor to maintain temperature. It is advisable to time trials using a stopwatch. Food should be placed into the proper goal zone using stainless steel tweezers if the study involves rewards.

Parameters Measured

1. **Latency to enter specific zones:** The time taken for a Zebrafish to enter a predefined zone of the maze after being introduced is used to assess exploratory behavior and the initial response to the environment. Shorter latencies may indicate higher exploratory behavior or lower anxiety.
2. **Time spent in specific zones:** The total amount of time a Zebrafish spends in different zones of the maze helps to determine zone preferences, which can be indicative of anxiety levels or exploratory tendencies. For example, more time spent in the periphery might suggest anxiety-like behavior.
3. **Distance traveled:** The total distance covered by the Zebrafish while exploring the maze reflects general locomotor activity and exploratory behavior. Increased distance can indicate higher activity levels or reduced anxiety.
4. **Number of entries into specific zones:** The number of times a Zebrafish enters different zones of the maze indicates the frequency of zone transitions, which can be related to exploratory behavior and willingness to explore new areas.
5. **Path taken (Trajectory):** It is the specific route taken by the Zebrafish through the maze. Analyzing the trajectory helps in understanding movement patterns, spatial learning, and decision-making processes.
6. **Thigmotaxis (Wall-hugging):** It is the tendency of the Zebrafish to stay close to the walls of the maze. Increased thigmotaxis is often interpreted as anxiety-like behavior. It reflects a preference for safer, enclosed areas over open spaces.
7. **Rearing and other vertical movements:** Vertical movements such as rearing (raising the body towards the surface) provide additional insights into exploratory behavior and anxiety. More vertical activity may indicate lower anxiety levels.
8. **Freezing behavior:** Periods of immobility, where the Zebrafish remains still, are referred to as freezing. Freezing is typically considered an indicator of fear or anxiety. Frequent or prolonged freezing suggests elevated levels of anxiety [3].

REQUIREMENTS

Animal: Adult Zebrafish

Equipment: Square-maze, ANY-maze, Camera, Graph-pad-prism.

PROCEDURE

1. The experiment begins by inducing a condition in the fish that may lead to cognitive impairments.
2. After the disease is introduced, the fish are placed in the first section of the SCM, and the time it takes them to reach the fourth section is recorded.
3. This process is repeated multiple times, and the average time is calculated. If the fish's cognitive abilities are intact, they will quickly learn the location of the reward and navigate to the fourth section of the maze in a short amount of time.
4. However, if their cognition has been altered due to the sickness, it will take them longer to reach their destination.
5. In addition to recording the time it takes for the fish to reach the reward, the time they spend in the fourth section is also recorded.
6. This is because cognitive impairments may cause the fish to have difficulty remembering the location of the reward or recognizing it as a desirable outcome.
7. Moreover, the SCM provides a reliable and efficient method for investigating potential cognitive flaws in the Zebrafish model.
8. By measuring the time it takes for the fish to navigate the maze and reach the reward, researchers can gain insights into the fish's cognitive abilities and potential cognitive impairments.

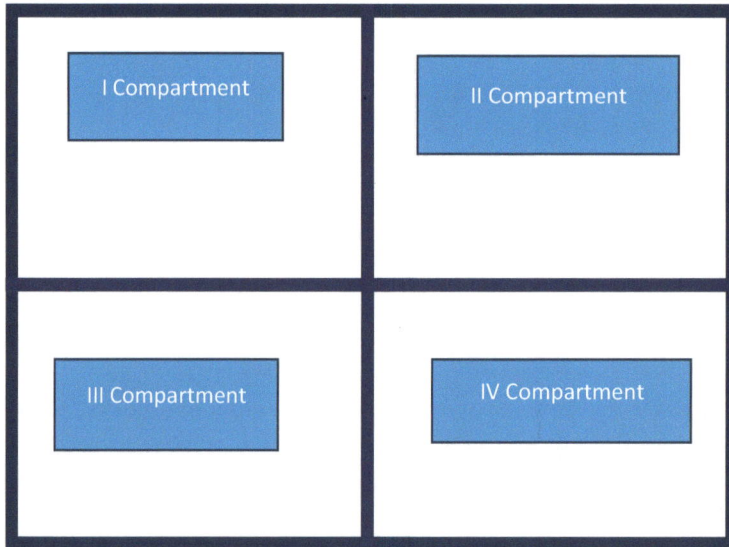

Fig. (14.1). Diagrammatic illustrations of square maze.

Data analysis: Data collected from the square maze test can be analyzed using statistical methods to identify patterns and correlations between behavioral responses, physiological parameters, and experimental conditions.

OBSERVATION

A dummy analysis is given in Table **14.1**.

Table 14.1. Observation table of escape latency and % of time spent in target quadrants on the square-maze apparatus by Zebrafish.

S. No.	Escape Latency(sec)	% Time Spent in the Target Quadrant
1.	180	65
2.	110	63
3.	126	76
4.	135	82
5.	141	59
Mean	138.4±26.02	69±9.6

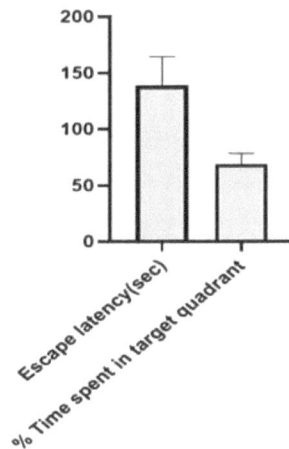

Statistical analysis: Statistical analysis shows a significant increase in escape latency as compared to the time spent in the target quadrant.

RESULT

The square maze test was performed, and the time was recorded successfully. The graph demonstrates a significant increase in escape latency as compared to the time spent in the target quadrant.

APPLICATIONS

Behavioral Insights

1. **Anxiety and exploration:** The square maze is particularly effective in assessing anxiety-like behaviors (*e.g.*, thigmotaxis or wall-hugging) and exploratory behavior.
2. **Learning and memory:** By introducing specific tasks or rewards, the maze can be used to evaluate cognitive functions such as spatial learning and memory retention.

Visual and Spatial Cues

1. **Environmental enrichment:** The maze can be enriched with visual and spatial cues to create more complex environments for cognitive and behavioral studies.
2. **Real-world relevance:** The use of such cues can help simulate more naturalistic settings, enhancing the ecological validity of the findings.

ADVANTAGES

Versatility

1. **Multiple behavior assessed:** The square maze can be used to study a range of behaviors, including exploration, anxiety, learning, and memory.
2. **Adaptability:** The maze can be modified to suit different experimental designs and objectives, such as adding barriers or zones to create different task complexities.

Quantifiable Measures

1. **Clear metrics:** Researchers can easily quantify behaviors such as latency to enter zones, time spent in zones, distance traveled, and the number of zone entries.
2. **Automated tracking:** The use of video tracking software allows for precise and objective measurement of Zebrafish movements and behaviours.

Standardization

1. **Consistency:** The square maze provides a consistent and controlled environment for behavioral testing, reducing variability and improving the reliability of results.
2. **Reproducibility:** Standardized protocols for the square maze ensure that experiments can be replicated across different labs and studies.

Ease of Use

1. **Simple setup:** The square maze is relatively easy to set up and use, making it accessible for researchers at various levels of expertise.
2. **Low cost:** Constructing a square maze is cost-effective, and it can be made from inexpensive materials like acrylic or glass.

Non-invasive Observation

1. **Minimal stress:** The square maze allows for non-invasive observation of Zebrafish behavior, minimizing stress and potential harm to the animals.
2. **Ethical considerations:** Non-invasive methods align with ethical standards for animal research, promoting animal welfare.

Applicability to High-Throughput Screening

1. **Multiple animals:** Multiple Zebrafish can be tested simultaneously in separate mazes or compartments, enabling high-throughput screening of behaviors.
2. **Drug testing:** The maze is suitable for pharmacological studies, allowing researchers to assess the effects of drugs on behavior in a systematic manner.

LIMITATIONS

Limited Naturalistic Environment

1. **Behavioral relevance:** Square mazes do not closely replicate the natural habitats of Zebrafish, which are typically more complex and structurally varied. As a result, this may lead to less ecologically valid outcomes.
2. **Stress induction:** The unnatural environment can induce stress in Zebrafish, potentially affecting their behavior and confounding the results.

Spatial Constraints

1. **Movement restriction:** The corners and straight edges of a square maze can limit the natural swimming patterns of Zebrafish, which might prefer more fluid and curved trajectories.
2. **Exploration limitation:** Zebrafish may explore a square maze less thoroughly than a more naturally designed environment, potentially skewing the data on exploration and spatial learning.

Data Interpretation

1. **Ambiguous results:** Interpreting the data from a square maze can be challenging. For instance, it might be difficult to differentiate between thigmotaxis (wall-hugging behavior) due to anxiety and genuine spatial

exploration.
2. **Corner behavior:** Zebrafish might spend disproportionate amounts of time in the corners of the maze, which can be interpreted differently depending on the experimental context (*e.g.*, as a sign of anxiety or preference).

Experimental Control

1. **Lighting and reflection:** The shape and structure of a square maze can lead to uneven lighting and reflections, which might affect Zebrafish behavior. Controlling these variables can be challenging.
2. **Water flow dynamics:** Square mazes may create non-uniform water flow patterns, affecting the Zebrafish's movement and potentially influencing the outcomes of the study.

Limited Task Variety

1. **Cognitive testing:** Square mazes may not be suitable for a broad range of cognitive and behavioral tests. For instance, complex tasks that require more intricate navigation and problem-solving may be better suited to mazes with more varied layouts.
2. **Learning and memory:** Studies on learning and memory might be constrained by the simplistic design of a square maze, which may not offer enough complexity to challenge the Zebrafish adequately.

Comparison with other Models

1. **Benchmarking issues:** If the goal is to compare results with studies using other maze designs (*e.g.*, circular or T-mazes), the differences in maze structure can complicate direct comparisons and meta-analyses.
2. **Species-specificity:** The square maze might not be the best model for all species, making it less versatile for comparative studies involving multiple types of fish or other aquatic organisms.

PRACTICE QUESTIONS

1. What is the primary objective of using a square maze in this study?
2. How does the square maze design fit the specific research question or hypothesis?
3. What measures are in place to minimize stress for the Zebrafish in the square maze?
4. What specific behaviors are being measured in the square maze?
5. How will the data be collected and analyzed to differentiate between exploration, anxiety, and other behaviors?

REFERENCES

[1]   Meshalkina DA, Kizlyk MN, Kysil EV, *et al.* Understanding zebrafish cognition. Behav Processes 2017; 141(Pt 2): 229-41.
[http://dx.doi.org/10.1016/j.beproc.2016.11.020] [PMID: 27919782]

[2]   Collier AD, Khan KM, Caramillo EM, Mohn RS, Echevarria DJ. Zebrafish and conditioned place preference: A translational model of drug reward. Prog Neuropsychopharmacol Biol Psychiatry 2014; 55: 16-25.
[http://dx.doi.org/10.1016/j.pnpbp.2014.05.014] [PMID: 24887295]

[3]   Silva PF, de Leaniz CG, Luchiari AC. Fear contagion in zebrafish: A behaviour affected by familiarity. BioRxiv. 2019: 521187.

CHAPTER 15

Novel Object Recognition Task in Zebrafish

Dhrita Chatterjee[1] and Shamsher Singh[1,*]

[1] *Neuropharmacology Division, Department of Pharmacology, ISF College of Pharmacy, Moga, Punjab 142001, India*

INTRODUCTION

Aim: The aim of this chapter is to investigate the memory and cognition of Zebrafish, a freshwater teleost, using a novel object recognition test (NORT).

Scope and outcomes: Through this practical technique, we can analyze the memory recognition and cognitive abilities of a fish by observing their preference for choosing and retaining a new object over a familiar object. This study provides insights into the fish's ability to recognize and remember new objects as well as to study their learning capabilities. By performing the test, researchers can better understand how various environmental and genetic factors influence the cognition of the fish.

Theory: The Novel Object Recognition (NOR) test has become an increasingly important method for evaluating learning and memory in Zebrafish, similar to rodents. In 1988, Ennaceur and Delacour first described the NOR test, primarily using rats. This test examines the ability of a fish to explore more frequently toward a new object than a familiar one. Consequently, a stronger preference towards unfamiliar objects indicates memory recognition and consolidation.

The NOR test is a quick and attractive method that requires no reward or punishment; instead, only minimal training or habituation is necessary. This test is very useful for assessing long-term, intermediate, and short-term memory by adjusting the retention interval. Basically, maze and open field apparatus are used for performing the NOR test in both fish and rodents. Ennaceur and Delacour (1988) used a wooden open box measuring 65 × 45 × 65 cm (Fig. **15.1**) [1].

* **Corresponding author Shamsher Singh:** Neuropharmacology Division, Department of Pharmacology, ISF College of Pharmacy, Moga, Punjab 142001, India; Tel: +91-9779980588; E-mail: shamshersinghbajwa@gmail.com

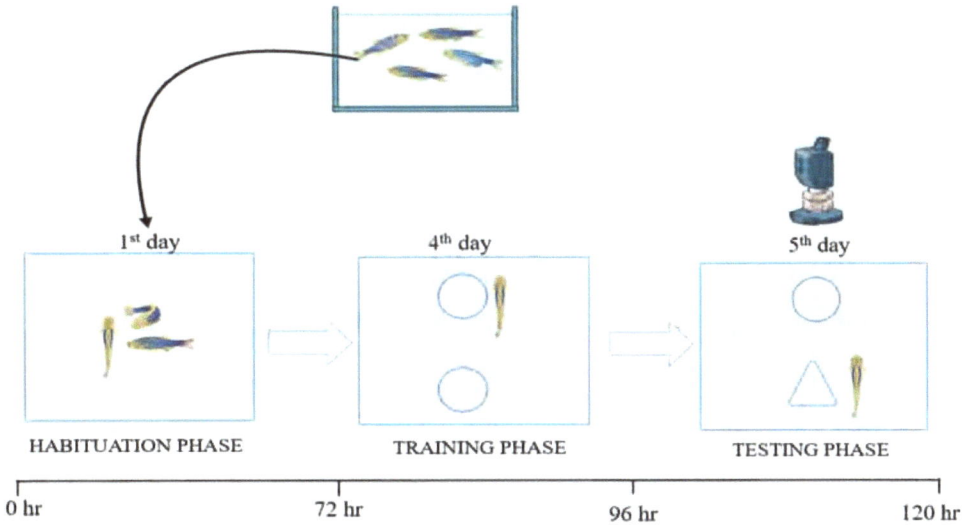

Fig. (15.1). In this picture, three sessions of novel object recognition test (NORT) are shown.

In contrast, Zebrafish were tested in 15L tanks measuring 29cm × 14cm × 18cm. Fishes were kept in the holding tanks in between trials and exposed to the experimental tanks containing the objects. Both tanks have similar dimensions. The novelty of performing the NOR test is to determine the recognition memory of fish. It is a highly validated test used to assess the effectiveness of drugs that improve memory, the (negative) impact of other substances on memory, or the impact of aging or heredity on memory [2].

REQUIREMENTS

Animal: Adult Zebrafish

Equipment: Novel Object Recognition test apparatus, Any maze software, Graph pad prism, Camera.

PROCEDURE

The NOR test requires only three sessions: (1) Habituation session, (2) Training session, (3) Testing session

1. During the habituation phase, remove the fish from the holding tank and expose it in the central portion of the experimental tank.
2. Make sure that the procedure is carried out in a quiet environment, and the temperature of the water should be maintained.
3. In the absence of objects, allow the fish to move freely throughout the

experimental tank for at least 5 minutes to reduce novelty stress.
4. Then, return the fish to the holding tank. The habituation session continues for 3 days.
5. On the 4th day, place two identical objects inside the test tank, and the training session starts after exposing individual fish to the tank for 10 minutes.
6. Objects are either cube (side = 1.5 cm), round (5 mm), or sphere (diameter 3 cm). After 10 minutes of training, return the fish to the holding tank.
7. In the testing session, place one familiar object from the training session and replace the other with a new object, and then expose the fish in the experimental tank.
8. Allow the fish to move between these familiar and unfamiliar objects for around and check which object it prefers mostly.

During these 10 mins of the novel object recognition test, all behaviors of the fish are captured using a webcam that is connected to a laptop for further evaluation *via* the Any-Maze video-tracking system [3].

$$\%Preference = \frac{\text{Time of exploration to the novel object} \times 100}{\text{Time of exploration to the familial object} + \text{Time of exploration to the novel object}}$$

Conditions of the Environment

Water quality: To prevent any confusing stimuli, make sure the water remains consistently clean.

Water temperature: The optimal water temperature range is between 25.5 and 28.5 °C, and a 25-watt heater is placed at the bottom of the maze to maintain temperature. It is advisable to time trials using a stopwatch [4].

Data analysis: The data collected from the diving test can be analyzed using statistical methods to identify patterns and correlations between behavioral responses, physiological parameters, and experimental conditions.

OBSERVATION

The observation parameter (Dummy analysis) is described in Table **15.1**.

Table 15.1. Observation table of no. of entries and time of exploration on NORT of Zebrafish.

Fish No.	No. of Entries to Familiar Objects	Time of Exploration of the Familial Object (Sec)	No. of Entries to the New Object	Time of Exploration of the New Object (Sec)	% Preference
1.	8	65	18	62	48%
2.	12	75	9	79	51%

(Table 15.1) cont.....

Fish No.	No. of Entries to Familiar Objects	Time of Exploration of the Familial Object (Sec)	No. of Entries to the New Object	Time of Exploration of the New Object (Sec)	% Preference
3.	9	75	15	58	43%
4.	11	60	18	98	62%
Mean	10±1.8	68.7±7.5	15±4.2	74.2±18.26	51±8.04

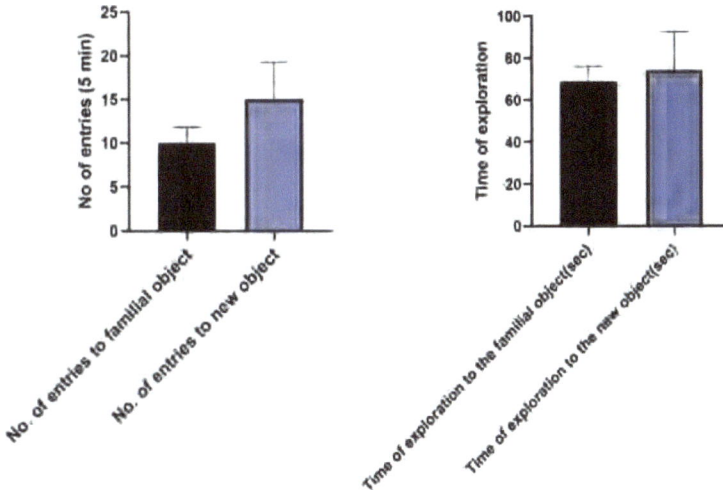

Statistical Analysis: Statistical analysis shows that the number of entries and the duration of exploration of the new object increase compared to those of the familiar object.

RESULT

The Novel Object Recognition (NOR) test was successfully conducted using adult zebrafish, with careful analysis of the results. The data, as presented in the observation table, were compared based on the number of entries and the duration of exploration for both familiar and unfamiliar objects. The graph demonstrates a significant increase in both the number of entries and the time spent exploring the unfamiliar object.

APPLICATIONS

1. **Disease identification:** The NOR test is used to evaluate various neurodegenerative disorders like Alzheimer's disease (AD), Parkinson's disease (PD), Huntington's disease (HD), *etc.*
2. **Evaluation of cognitive abilities:** It represents a wide range of applications not only for evaluating the pharmacological use of a drug but also for

characterizing the brain parts that are essential for various aspects of learning and memory.
3. **Drug screening:** It is used for assessing the impact of various drugs on memory and recognition of animals.
4. **Recognition of memory:** This test is used for assessing long-term, short-term, and sensory memory by measuring their capabilities for preferring the novel object rather than the familial object [5].

ADVANTAGES

1. **Less experimental stress:** As the habituation session is completed, it helps to reduce the experimental stress of the animals.
2. **Minimal training required:** In contrast to other behavioral tests, which might need multiple training sessions, NOR is a test where only one training session is required.
3. **Time-saving:** Requires less timing compared to other memory tests and chances of errors are less.
4. **Assessment of interest**: The main advantage over others is that it depends upon the innate curiosity of animals towards novelty without the need for any external force or training.
5. **Assessment of memory:** The ORT's biological reliability is higher than any other memory test as its conditions seem equivalent to those that are used for evaluating human cognition.

LIMITATIONS

1. **Low sensitivity:** NOR tests have low susceptibility compared to other behavioral tests.
2. **Environmental conditions:** Temperature and excess noise may alter the results of the tests. Odor can also create confusion in recognizing the new object.
3. **Limited scope:** As only one training session is performed, it is difficult to assess possible variations in the rate of learning.
4. **Change required:** One frequent way for modification to ORT is to use a new location instead of novel items, which allows the assessment of spatial memory [6].

PRACTICE QUESTIONS

1. What are the ideal dimensions of the apparatus used for the NOR test in Zebrafish?
2. What are the possible applications of the NOR test in fish?
3. What are the 3 phases involved in performing NOR test in fish?

4. What are the advantages of performing NOR in Zebrafish?

5. In the NOR test, which parts of the brain are potentially involved?

6. Describe in brief the procedure of NOR in fish.

REFERENCES

[1]   May Z, Morrill A, Holcombe A, *et al.* Object recognition memory in zebrafish. Behav Brain Res 2016; 296: 199-210.
      [http://dx.doi.org/10.1016/j.bbr.2015.09.016] [PMID: 26376244]

[2]   Stefanello FV, Fontana BD, Ziani PR, Müller TE, Mezzomo NJ, Rosemberg DB. Exploring object discrimination in zebrafish: Behavioral performance and scopolamine-induced cognitive deficits at different retention intervals. Zebrafish 2019; 16(4): 370-8.
      [http://dx.doi.org/10.1089/zeb.2018.1703] [PMID: 31145046]

[3]   Gaspary KV, Reolon GK, Gusso D, Bonan CD. Novel object recognition and object location tasks in zebrafish: Influence of habituation and NMDA receptor antagonism. Neurobiol Learn Mem 2018; 155: 249-60.
      [http://dx.doi.org/10.1016/j.nlm.2018.08.005] [PMID: 30086397]

[4]   Leger M, Quiedeville A, Bouet V, *et al.* Object recognition test in mice. Nat Protoc 2013; 8(12): 2531-7.
      [http://dx.doi.org/10.1038/nprot.2013.155] [PMID: 24263092]

[5]   Antunes M, Biala G. The novel object recognition memory: Neurobiology, test procedure, and its modifications. Cogn Process 2012; 13(2): 93-110.
      [http://dx.doi.org/10.1007/s10339-011-0430-z] [PMID: 22160349]

[6]   Lueptow LM. Novel object recognition test for the investigation of learning and memory in mice. Journal of visualized experiments: JoVE. 2017 (126).

CHAPTER 16

Open Field Test in Zebrafish

Mayank Attri[1], Anupam Awasthi[1] and Shamsher Singh[1,*]

[1] *Neuropharmacology Division, Department of Pharmacology, ISF College of Pharmacy, Moga, Punjab 142001, India*

INTRODUCTION

Aim: The aim of this study is to study the locomotor activities of Zebrafish (*Danio rerio*) using open-field apparatus.

Scope and outcomes: The open field apparatus allows for the assessment of Zebrafish exploration (locomotion) and instances of freezing behavior. Both adult rodents and Zebrafish exhibit strong scototaxis (preference for dark environments over light ones) and thigmotaxis (preference for staying close to the walls). Zebrafish exhibit habituation responses like those of rodents, altering their exploratory behavior as they go across new habitats. Researchers would likely observe and record the number of times the lines are crossed by Zebrafish in 5 minutes, time spent on corners, mirror biting, and freezing behavior, which is recorded by using various tracking software such as ANY-maze, Zebra Lab, Bonze, *etc*. In addition, researchers may conduct histopathological studies to validate the preliminary findings from the open field apparatus (OFA) and provide definitive evidence of any abnormal alterations in various regions of the brain.

Theory: A standard method for evaluating Zebrafish behavior and motility is the open field apparatus test (with ideal dimensions of $30 \times 30 \times 30$ cm), typically made of glass or plastic (Fig. **16.1**). This test is used to assess locomotion, aversion, and anxiety-like responses by observing changes in the Zebrafish's preferred locations. Formerly, various rodent-based models were utilized to find novel neuroactive medications, especially in the field of neurology. These approaches are productive, yet they have significant drawbacks (such as being time-consuming, expensive, and low output), which substantially decrease the chances of finding novel drugs.

---

*Corresponding author Shamsher Singh: Neuropharmacology Division, Department of Pharmacology, ISF College of Pharmacy, Moga, Punjab 142001, India; Tel: +91-9779980588; E-mail: shamshersinghbajwa@gmail.com

In contrast to previous models, the modern Zebrafish-based model offers several advantages for improved drug discovery and preclinical screening. Recently, the OFT has been used to analyze the swimming and locomotion patterns of Zebrafish, demonstrating a few similarities in the ways that rodents and Zebrafish explore unfamiliar environments [1]. The OFT is an animal anxiety/locomotion analysis model based on how animals naturally respond to unexpected circumstances. It can reveal a range of behaviors, from increased anxiety, which manifests as avoidance behavior (*e.g.*, decreased exploration, increased freezing, and/or disorganized, erratic locomotion), to heightened activity associated with exploration, demonstrating the animal's ability to explore new areas [2, 3].

A shift in behavior that could be an indication of adaptability to the new environment comes after this initial phase. For instance, as they get used to their new environment, the study subjects often decrease their mobility and develop an assortment of comfort behaviors. Also, the researchers might immensely benefit from the usage of OFA in hopes of accomplishing a spectrum of ground-breaking outcomes, such as executing novel research on links between numerous degenerative neurological conditions with specific newly discovered molecules, medicines, toxins, and chemicals.

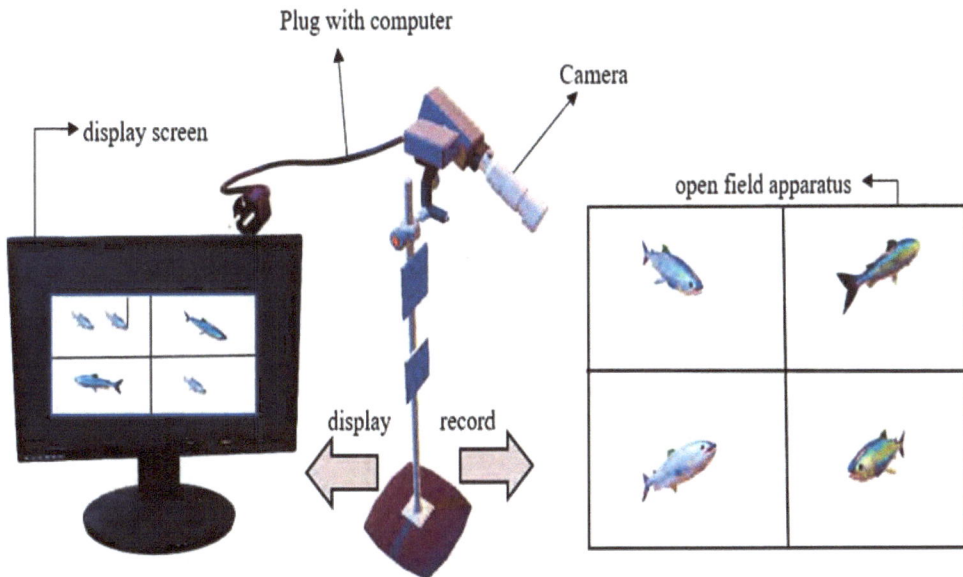

Fig. (16.1). Illustration of open-field apparatus.

REQUIREMENTS

Animal: Adult Zebrafish

Equipment: Open field apparatus, Any maze software, Graph pad prism, Camera.

PROCEDURE

1. Healthy Zebrafish should be selected for the conduction of the experimentation. All the procedures should be conducted with ethical guidelines provided by CPCSEA (The Committee for the Purpose of Control and Supervision of Experiments on Animals).
2. Usually, for the conductance of the study, the groups are divided into Control *vs.* Disease *vs.* Treatment with equal ratio of Zebrafish in each group.
3. The afflicted (diseased) group receives toxin, whereas the control group of Zebrafish receives no toxin, and the intervention group receives the desired drug dose for treatment as per the requirement of the researcher (the control group is used as a reference to compare the results of diseased *vs.* treatment).
4. Training is provided for four to five days for five minutes each morning and evening before the experiment day so that the Zebrafish could get habitual to the apparatus.
5. The study groups must keep on fasting for about 30 to 40 minutes before the start of trials on the sixth day, that being the day of the experiment.
6. The following behavior characteristics are recorded after Zebrafish are moved to the arena for the open field test, where they have five minutes (cut-off time) to explore.
7. Several behavioral outputs that are measured include time spent in the arena's center, freezing behavior, thigmotaxis, no. of lines crossed, and mirror biting behavior, and then control *vs.* diseased *vs.* treatment groups are recorded and compared.
8. In the mirror biting test, Zebrafish interact with their mirror images, and the number of times a fish attacks its reflection during a five-minute period is used to specifically measure aggression.

OBSERVATION

The observation parameter (Dummy analysis) is described in Table **16.1**.

Table 16.1. Different parameters of open field test apparatus of Zebrafish.

S. No.	No. of Times Lines were Crossed in 5 Mins	Time Spent in Corners (Sec)	Freezing Behavior (Sec)	Mirror Biting
1.	8	120 sec	40 sec	12
2.	12	280sec	60 sec	10
3.	16	180sec	95sec	8

(Table 16.1) cont.....

S. No.	No. of Times Lines were Crossed in 5 Mins	Time Spent in Corners (Sec)	Freezing Behavior (Sec)	Mirror Biting
4.	18	200 sec	120 sec	6
Mean	13.5 ± 3.8	195 ± 57.2	78.75 ± 30.9	9.0 ± 2.2

Statistical analysis:

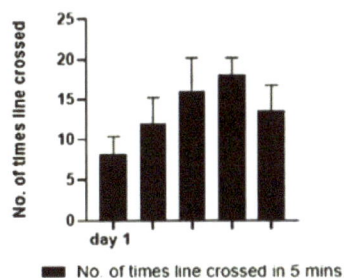

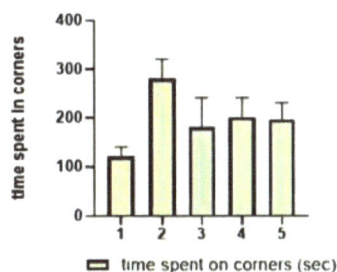

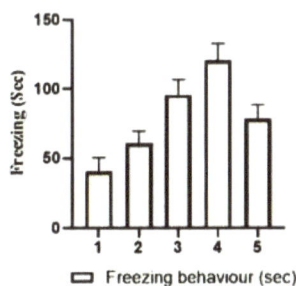

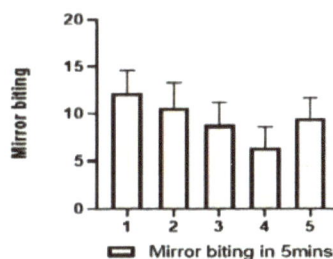

Statistical significance: The graphs show the significant difference in different parameters of open field apparatus.

RESULT

The open-field test apparatus parameters were studied and understood successfully. The results show the significant difference in different parameters of open field apparatus.

APPLICATIONS

1. The open field apparatus is generally used for the assessment of locomotion activity, exploration, and anxiety-related disorders.
2. To better understand the behaviors of the group that was treated to develop and

improve treatment options, animal groups in intervention or disease models might have their open-field task behaviors compared to a control group or a normal group of animals.

3. In addition to exposing Zebrafish to the novelty of an open-field arena, animals may be reintroduced to the arena and given habituation tasks. This approach allows for a more effective understanding of the animals' habituation behaviors.

4. The open field apparatus and Zebrafish are widely used for the study of various neurodegenerative diseases, which include Huntington's disease (hyperkinesia), Alzheimer's disease, Parkinson's disease (hypokinesia), epilepsy, traumatic brain injury, autism, and other neurological disorders that specifically alter locomotor activity, which were studied by using the open field apparatus.

5. The open field test is a simple and easily modifiable apparatus with a wide range of research applications, including aging, treatment effects, and lesions.

The Zebrafish has applications in various other fields, including:

1. Behavioral research
2. Toxicology
3. Oncology
4. Neurobehavioral
5. Reproductive studies
6. Teratogenicity studies
7. Genetics
8. Neurobiology

ADVANTAGES

1. Researchers will appreciate this innovative tool to conduct a variety of investigations for vibrant, innovative new results and discoveries.

2. The open field apparatus can also be used to gauge the degree of habituation to the novel environment simply because when utilized for prolonged periods of time, spontaneous motor behavior in the open field apparatus reduces, which is a sign of habituation.

3. Through open-field apparatus, numerous physiological effects, toxins, and neurodegenerative illnesses can be scrutinized.

4. Contrasted to many other apparatus, open field apparatus is more facile for researchers to utilize and comprehend for locomotion analysis.

5. An animal's level of spontaneous motor activity and exploratory behavior can be assessed through open-field analysis.

LIMITATIONS

1. Lack of training can alter Zebrafish's normal behavior.
2. Excessive stress given to studying subjects may create variations in observations.
3. Zebrafish require attention all the time.
4. Open-field apparatus does not specifically differentiate between fear and anxiety-like behavior.
5. Numerous environmental factors, such as water properties (*e.g.*, pH, temperature) and even noise levels around the apparatus, can impact the outcomes. To ensure the reliability and consistency of the data, these factors must be carefully controlled.

PRACTICE QUESTIONS

- What must the apparatus's ideal dimension be?
- If the apparatus's dimensions are increased to provide the study subject (rodent) additional room to move around, will this have an impact on anxiety or locomotion behavior?
- What are the various studies that are conducted using open-field apparatus and Zebrafish?
- Differentiating fear and anxiety?
- What are open-field apparatus water quality parameters?

REFERENCES

[1]   Scatterty KR, Pitman T, Eckersley T, Schmaltz R, Hamilton TJ. Zebrafish aversion to infrasound in an open field test. Front Behav Neurosci 2023; 16: 1019368.
[http://dx.doi.org/10.3389/fnbeh.2022.1019368] [PMID: 36688130]

[2]   Midttun HLE, Vindas MA, Nadler LE, Øverli Ø, Johansen IB. Behavioural effects of the common brain-infecting parasite *Pseudoloma neurophilia* in laboratory zebrafish (*Danio rerio*). Sci Rep 2020; 10(1): 8083.
[http://dx.doi.org/10.1038/s41598-020-64948-8] [PMID: 32415102]

[3]   Godwin J, Sawyer S, Perrin F, Oxendine SE, Kezios ZD. Adapting the open field test to assess anxiety-related behavior in Zebrafish. In: Kalueff A, Stewart A, Eds. Zebrafish protocols for neurobehavioral research Neuromethods. Totowa, NJ: Humana Press 2012; 66.
[http://dx.doi.org/10.1007/978-1-61779-597-8_13]

CHAPTER 17

T-Maze Test in Zebrafish

Kousik Maparu[1], Vaishali[1], Dilpreet Kaur[1] and Shamsher Singh[1,*]

[1] *Neuropharmacology Division, Department of Pharmacology, ISF College of Pharmacy, Moga, Punjab 142001, India*

INTRODUCTION

Aim: The aim of this study is to check the memory function of an adult Zebrafish by using a T-maze apparatus.

Scope and Outcomes: T-maze is behavioral activity testing equipment widely used to study exploratory behavior in animals such as rodents and Zebrafish, particularly in the context of the central nervous system (CNS). It is employed to assess memory function, spatial learning activities, depression, and anxiety-related behavior. By conducting this experiment, researchers can gain valuable insights into how genetic and environmental factors influence cognitive functions in animals.

Theory: The T-maze apparatus consists of three arms: a main arm that brunches into two secondary arms, typically differentiated by colored markers. The arms are covered with colored paper: red to indicate a "stressed" arm and green to signify a "relaxed" arm [1]. The apparatus is usually constructed from Plexiglas and is available in various sizes and configurations to suit experimental models.

A range of experimental protocols can be applied with T-maze. For instance, researchers can evaluate visual discrimination by designating specific target zones or enrichment chambers within the maze's arm using colored or patterned sleeves. Environmental enrichment or food rewards may be placed in the goal zone to provide positive reinforcement during the test.

Although the proportions can be changed, we advise selecting a maze design that is either a symmetrical-shaped configuration (50 cm x 50 cm x 10 cm) or a cross-

---

* **Corresponding author Shamsher Singh:** Neuropharmacology Division, Department of Pharmacology, ISF College of Pharmacy, Moga, Punjab 142001, India; Tel: +91-9779980588; E-mail: shamshersinghbajwa@gmail.com

shaped configuration (70 cm x 50 cm x 10 cm) (Fig. **17.1**). It is best to utilize detachable opaque Plexiglas doors to keep the maze's arms separated from the goal and start zones. Make sure the arms of the maze are closed off from the goal and start zones with Plexiglas doors [2].

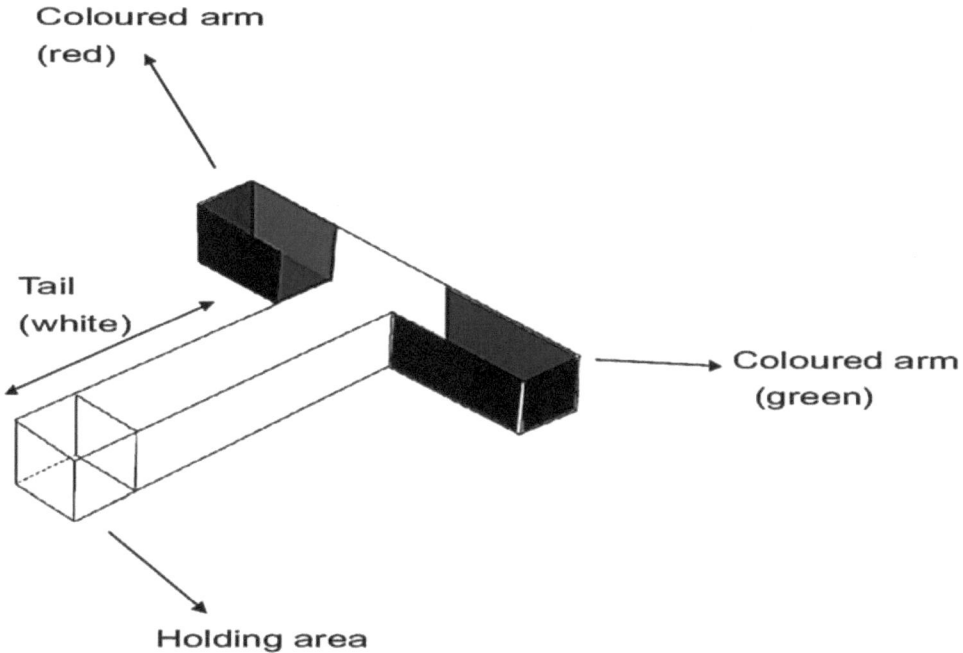

Fig. (**17.1**). Diagram illustrating the T-maze apparatus.

REQUIREMENTS

Animal: Adult Zebrafish

Equipment: T-maze, ANY-maze, Camera, Graph-pad-prism.

PROCEDURE

The T-maze apparatus has three phases, including the habituation phase, the training phase, and the testing phase.

1. The Zebrafish is allowed to freely explore the maze for 5 minutes during the initial habituation phase.
2. The Zebrafish is then introduced into the main arm of the maze for 2 minutes.
3. After 2 minutes, the Zebrafish is gently guided toward the red chamber, which is then closed with a glass lid.

4. In the red chamber, the Zebrafish is exposed for 5 minutes, during which time it is gently stimulated using a glass rod to introduce irritation in the Zebrafish.
5. After 5 minutes, Zebrafish is pushed toward the green-colored chamber for 5 minutes, where it is rewarded with feed.
6. This activity is performed three or more times for habituation and training to reduce handling and novelty stress.
7. In the training phase, follow the same procedure as in the habituation phase and conduct training trials 2 times at an interval of 24 hours.
8. In the testing phase, follow the same procedure as in the trial phase, and after the testing session, return the fish to its home tank [3].
9. In the testing phase, observe the effect of the drug on the learning and memory behavior in Zebrafish and count the number of entries and time spent on each arm.

Conditions of the Environment

Water Quality: To prevent any confusing stimuli, make sure the water is consistently clean.

Water Temperature: Fill the maze with either tank water or a combination of tank water and filtered tap water that has been treated with conditioner up to a height of around 8 to 10 cm. The ideal water temperature range is between 25.5 and 28.5 °C, and a 25-watt heater is placed on the maze's floor to maintain temperature. It is advisable to time trials using a stopwatch. Food should be placed into the proper goal zone using stainless steel tweezers if the study involves rewards [4].

OBSERVATION

A dummy analysis is given in Table **17.1**.

Table 17.1. No. of entry and time spent in different zones on the T-maze apparatus of Zebrafish.

S. No.	No. of Entry in the Red Zone	Time spent in the Red Zone (Sec.)	No. of entry in the Green Zone	Time spent in the Green Zone (Sec.)
01	2	30	3	112
02	3	26	5	98
03	2	25	3	147
04	3	37	5	182
05	4	29	4	128
Mean	2.8±0.8	29.40±2.11	4.0±1.0	133.4±14.64

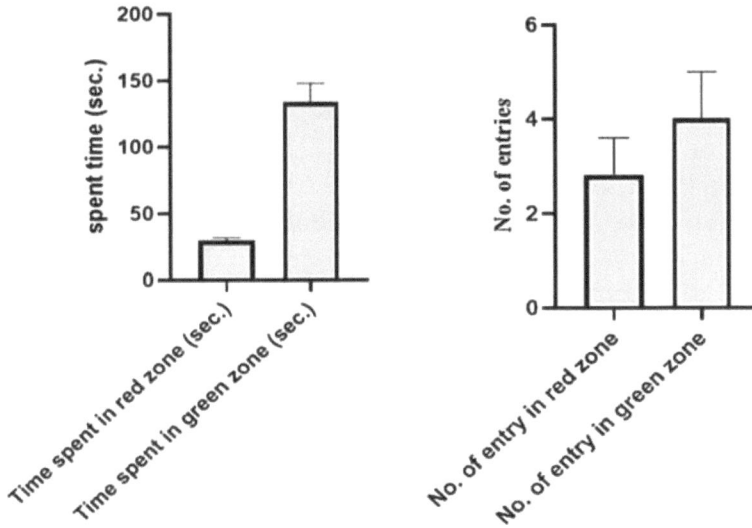

Statistical analysis: Statistical analysis shows a significant increase in time spent and the number of entries in the green zone as compared to the red zone.

RESULT

The T-maze test using Zebrafish was performed successfully using adult Zebrafish. The data, as represented in the observation table, were compared based on the time spent and the number of entries in the red zone as well green zone. The graph demonstrates a significant increase in time spent and the number of entries in the green zone as compared to the red zone.

APPLICATIONS

1. **Disease identification:** The T-maze test is used to evaluate various neurodegenerative disorders like Alzheimer's disease (AD), Parkinson's disease (PD), Huntington's disease (HD), *etc*.
2. **Evaluation of cognitive abilities:** It represents a wide range of applications not only for evaluating the pharmacological use of a drug but also for characterizing the brain parts that are essential for various aspects of learning and memory.
3. **Drug screening:** It is used for assessing the impact of various drugs on memory and recognition of animals.
4. **Recognition of memory:** This test is used for assessing long-term, short-term, and sensory memory by measuring their capabilities for preferring the novel object rather than the familiar object [5].

ADVANTAGES

1. **Less experimental stress:** As the habituation session is completed, it helps to reduce the experimental stress of the animals.
2. **Relevance to Human Models:** The Zebrafish T-maze provides a cost-effective, high-throughput model to study learning and memory, closely mirroring human cognitive processes. Its conserved neurobiological pathways enable translational insights into neurodegenerative diseases like Alzheimer's.
3. **Assessment of interest:** The main advantage over others is that it depends upon the innate curiosity of animals towards novelty without the need for any external force or training.
4. **Minimal instruction needed:** Zebrafish may react to their mirror without requiring a great deal of instruction. The test is easy to administer as there is a strong and quick natural reaction to a perceived conspecific.
5. **Versatility:** Aside from anxiety, a broad variety of behaviors, including exploration, novelty seeking, and risk assessment, may be studied using the plus maze. It is a widely valuable tool in behavioral neuroscience because of its adaptability [6].

LIMITATIONS

1. **Environmental sensitivity:** Several environmental elements, including illumination, water quality, and tank configuration, may have an impact on Zebrafish behavior in the plus maze. Strict standardization is necessary for this sensitivity to guarantee consistency and repeatability in the outcomes.
2. **Stress induction:** If the lighting is excessively bright or there are quick changes between open and closed arms, the test setting itself may cause stress. The perception of behavior associated with worry may get confused by this stress.
3. **Synthetic environment:** The plus maze is a synthetic setting that could not accurately reflect the natural circumstances that Zebrafish encounter in the wild. This may reduce the results' ecological validity and their suitability for natural behaviors [7].

PRACTICE QUESTIONS

1. What are the ideal dimensions of the apparatus used for the T-maze test in Zebrafish?
2. What are the advantages of performing T-maze in Zebrafish?
3. What are the 3 phases involved in performing a T-maze test in Zebrafish?
4. In the T-maze test, which parts of the brain are potentially involved?
5. Describe in brief the procedure of T-maze in Zebrafish.
6. What are the possible applications of the T-maze test in Zebrafish?

REFERENCES

[1]   Ali M. An Assessment of Zebrafish natural color preference and its modification by stimuli, 2018.

[2]   Ngoc Hieu BT, Ngoc Anh NT, Audira G, *et al.* Development of a modified three-day T-maze protocol for evaluating learning and memory capacity of adult zebrafish. Int J Mol Sci 2020; 21(4): 1464.
[http://dx.doi.org/10.3390/ijms21041464] [PMID: 32098080]

[3]   Shoji H, Hagihara H, Takao K, Hattori S, Miyakawa T. T-maze forced alternation and left-right discrimination tasks for assessing working and reference memory in mice. J Vis Exp 2012; (60): e3300.
[PMID: 22395674]

[4]   Peitsaro N, Kaslin J, Anichtchik OV, Panula P. Modulation of the histaminergic system and behaviour by α-fluoromethylhistidine in zebrafish. J Neurochem 2003; 86(2): 432-41.
[http://dx.doi.org/10.1046/j.1471-4159.2003.01850.x] [PMID: 12871584]

[5]   Wu CY, Lerner FM, Silva ACE, *et al.* Utilizing the modified T-maze to assess functional memory outcomes after cardiac arrest. Journal of visualized experiments: JoVE. 2018(131).

[6]   Vignet C, Bégout ML, Péan S, Lyphout L, Leguay D, Cousin X. Systematic screening of behavioral responses in two zebrafish strains. Zebrafish 2013; 10(3): 365-75.
[http://dx.doi.org/10.1089/zeb.2013.0871] [PMID: 23738739]

CHAPTER 18

Learning Test in Zebrafish

Romanpreet Kaur[1] and **Shamsher Singh**[1,*]

[1] *Neuropharmacology Division, Department of Pharmacology, ISF College of Pharmacy, Moga, Punjab 142001, India*

INTRODUCTION

Aim: The aim of this chapter is to perform the learning test in Zebrafish.

Scope and outcomes: The learning test is a behavioral activity test for analyzing exploratory behavior regarding central nervous system (CNS) disorders across various species like rodents and Zebrafish. It is used to study memory function and spatial learning activities, depression, and anxiety behavior.

Theory: To evaluate Zebrafish's cognitive abilities, specifically their capacity for learning and memory, a learning test is used. The goal of these tests is to assess the fish's capacity for learning and memory related to tasks, like rewarding a stimulus or avoiding a certain location after a bad experience. Measurements of the fish's behavior and performance over time are made in controlled environments, including tanks with characteristics or mazes.

Novelty in learning tests with Zebrafish often involves assessing their responses to new environments or stimuli. Apart from assessing anxiety and stress responses, these tests can also evaluate traumatic brain injury (TBI) in Zebrafish.

TYPES OF LEARNING

Zebrafish demonstrate various forms of learning, such as:

Non-associative learning

1. **Habituation:** A decrease in the response to a repeated stimulus, such as a reduced startle response to a sound that is presented repeatedly.
2. **Sensitization:** An increased sensitivity and heightened locomotor activity following repeated exposure to a stimulus, such as nicotine, leading to a more pronounced response with subsequent exposures.

* **Corresponding author Shamsher Singh:** Neuropharmacology Division, Department of Pharmacology, ISF College of Pharmacy, Moga, Punjab 142001, India; Tel: +91-9779980588; E-mail: shamshersinghbajwa@gmail.com

Associative Learning

Classical (Pavlovian) Conditioning

1. **Appetitive conditioning:** An enhancement or attenuation of a reflexive response after the association of a cue with a favorable stimulus.
2. **Aversive conditioning:** An enhancement or attenuation of a reflexive response after the association of a cue with an unfavorable stimulus.

Operant (Instrumental) Conditioning

1. **Positive reinforcement:** An increased response to obtain an appetitive stimulus, such as approaching a sensor that dispenses food.
2. **Negative reinforcement:** An enhancement in response to removing an unpleasant stimulus, such as entering a section without shock upon encountering a light previously associated with shock.
3. **Positive punishment:** A reduction in response after the association of behavior with an unpleasant stimulus.
4. **Negative punishment:** A reduction in response after the attribution of behaviors to the absence of an appetitive stimulus.

Other Types of Learning

1. **Social (shoaling) learning:** Groups of Zebrafish exhibit faster learning rates compared to individuals.
2. **Motor learning:** Zebrafish adjust their locomotor commands using sensory feedback to perform accurate movements, thereby enhancing accuracy and coordination.

Behavioral Learning in Zebrafish

Like many other animals, Zebrafish acquire new behaviors through experience and contact with their surroundings. This process is known as behavioral learning. Because of their transparent larvae, which allow researchers to see their brain activity in real time, and relatively basic neural circuitry, Zebrafish are particularly fascinating subjects for studying behavioral learning. These are some significant aspects of Zebrafish behavioral learning, such as associative learning, spatial learning, social learning, habituation, sensitization, operant conditioning, and neural mechanisms.

Research on behavioral learning in Zebrafish offers valuable insights into the fundamental principles of learning and memory across a variety of species, including humans. It also enhances our understanding of the cognitive abilities of Zebrafish, providing a comparative framework for studying learning processes in more complex organisms [1].

Behavioral Learning in Various Diseases

The study of behavioral learning in Zebrafish has been examined for several illnesses, especially those that impact behavior and brain function. Several notable examples consist of:

1. **Autism spectrum disorders (ASD):** Zebrafish's social nature and capacity to pick up on socially significant cues have made them useful models for several aspects of ASD. Scientists have investigated the effects of ASD-related gene mutations on Zebrafish's social interaction, communication, and learning.
2. **Epilepsy:** To investigate seizure behavior and its underlying causes, Zebrafish models of epilepsy have been created. In addition to testing possible antiepileptic medications, researchers utilize these models to study how seizures impact Zebrafish learning and memory functions.
3. **Alzheimer's disease:** Alzheimer's disease-related cognitive abnormalities, such as learning and memory problems, have been studied using Zebrafish. Models of transgenic Zebrafish that exhibit mutations in the tau or amyloid-beta proteins have been used to study prospective treatment approaches and disease processes.
4. **Parkinson's disease:** Parkinson's disease-affected Zebrafish models show motor deficits like human symptoms. Additionally, studies have examined how learning and cognitive processes are affected in these models by mutations linked to Parkinson's disease.
5. **Fragile X syndrome:** Fragile X syndrome is a genetic condition linked to intellectual incapacity and behavioral difficulties. It has been studied using Zebrafish. Researchers investigated altered behavior and learning deficits in Zebrafish models with mutations in genes associated with fragile X.
6. **Drug addiction:** The behavioral impact of substances of abuse and behaviors connected to addiction has been studied using Zebrafish. Zebrafish models of drug-seeking behavior, reward processing, and behavioral sensitization can be evaluated by researchers, offering valuable insights into the brain circuits implicated in addiction.
7. **Anxiety and depression:** Models of Zebrafish have been used to investigate behaviors like depression and anxiety. Researchers investigate how stress responses, fear conditioning, and other behaviors associated with anxiety and depression are affected by genetic mutations or pharmacological interventions [2].

Researchers can investigate the underlying mechanisms of neurological and psychiatric diseases, particularly how these conditions affect behavior-learning processes, using these disease models in Zebrafish. Zebrafish is a useful tool for evaluating possible therapies and looking at advanced treatments for certain illnesses.

Instruments or Apparatus for Behavior Learning in Zebrafish

It takes specialized instruments and equipment to accurately monitor and measure the behavior of Zebrafish to study behavior learning in them. To investigate how Zebrafish acquire behavior, the following instruments are frequently used:

1. **Video tracking systems:** Video tracking technologies are necessary for automatically capturing and non-intrusively analyzing Zebrafish behavior. To record the fish's movements, these systems usually use cameras positioned above or around the experimental tank. These systems' software can measure things like swimming speed, distance traveled, preferred location, and response to stimuli.

2. **Automated behavioral assay systems:** These systems combine controlled surroundings with video tracking to perform behavioral tests. For example, the Zebra Box system establishes controlled environments for Zebrafish behavior studies, enabling scientists to evaluate the fishes' reactions to stimuli like changes in light and dark or the presence of predators.

3. **Multi-compartment tanks:** Multiple Zebrafish can be tested simultaneously in controlled environments due to the design of multi-compartment tanks. Studies on spatial learning, social behavior, or conditioned responses can be made easier with the help of these tanks, which may contain separators or distinct areas where various stimuli or circumstances can be presented.

4. **Optogenetics and chemogenetics equipment:** Zebrafish brain circuits are studied and manipulated using optogenetics and chemogenetics. Neuronal activity is modulated, and the effects on behavior learning are studied using tools like LED light sources for optogenetic stimulation and microinjection devices for delivering chemicals (like designer receptors exclusively activated by designer drugs or DREADDs).

5. **T-maze and Y-maze apparatus:** Zebrafish are tested using these mazes to evaluate their spatial learning and memory. Zebrafish are taught to navigate through spatial cues and select between many pathways linked to rewards or punishments using these two or three arms.

6. **Operant conditioning chambers:** Zebrafish operant behaviors and reward-based learning are studied in operant conditioning chambers. Zebrafish can interact with these chambers' potential touchscreens and levers to obtain rewards (such as food pellets) as a reward for doing particular tasks.

7. **Electrophysiology setup:** Electrical signals from the Zebrafish brain are recorded and analyzed using electrophysiological setups to examine the

neuronal activity underlying behavior learning. Microelectrodes or calcium imaging techniques are commonly used in these setups to track neuronal activity during behavioral tasks or in response to stimuli.

8. **Environmental control systems:** For behavior learning experiments, it is essential to maintain constant environmental settings. To reduce unpredictability and guarantee accurate experimental results, environmental control systems regulate variables, including temperature, lighting conditions (light/dark cycles), water quality (*e.g.*, pH, conductivity), and oxygen levels.

With the use of these instruments and setups, scientists may carry out complex studies to investigate all aspects of Zebrafish behavior learning, from simple associative learning to complicated social interactions and cognitive processes. They offer important insights into the genetic foundations and brain mechanisms underlying behavior learning in a variety of settings and circumstances.

APPARATUS

The apparatus used in Zebrafish learning testing includes:

T-MAZE TEST

A T-shaped maze is used to measure Zebrafish preference for novel locations or areas to evaluate their ability to recognize and remember spatial information. The T-maze is described in Fig. (**18.1**).

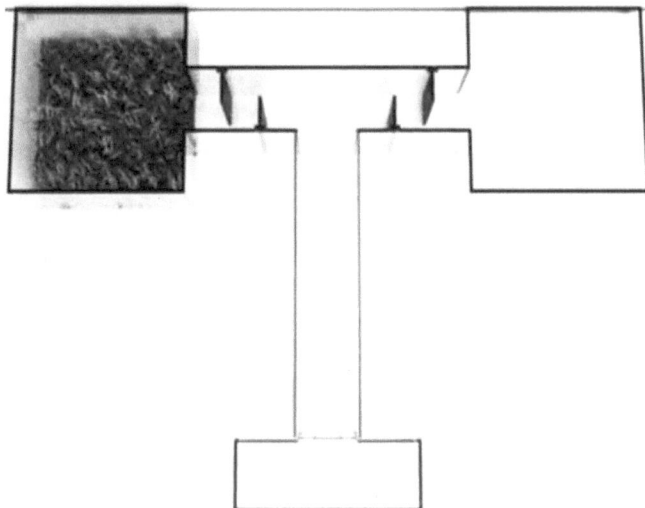

Fig. (18.1). T-maze test apparatus.

Requirements

Animal: Adult Zebrafish

Equipment: T-maze apparatus, Any maze software, Graph pad prism, Camera.

Procedure

1. There are several possible layouts for the maze, including symmetrical (50 cm x 50 cm x 10 cm) and cross (70 cm x 50 cm x 10 cm).
2. To reduce stress, Zebrafish are allowed to become familiar with the lab environment for a certain amount of time before the test.
3. Zebrafish are placed in a T-shaped maze featuring detachable opaque Plexiglas doors and a clear Plexiglas body. The fish are free to swim in the water that fills the maze.
4. By hiding food rewards in particular arms, the fish are trained to find their way around the maze. The layout of the maze forces the fish to make decisions to get to the food rewards, which enables the assessment of memory and learning.
5. A camera records the fish's behavior, and it measures how long it takes to get to the goal zone or what proportion of its decisions are right. This test is intended to evaluate the fish's capacity for learning and memory [3].

Observation

A dummy analysis is given in Table **18.1**.

Table 18.1. Observation table of No. of entries and time spent in different zones on the T-maze apparatus of Zebrafish.

Trial No.	No. of Entries		New Objects' Contact Time (Sec)	Total Duration of Time (Sec)
	Right Arm	Light Arm		
1.	3	2	20	31
2.	5	3	22	43
3.	3	2	25	35
4.	5	3	15	45
5.	4	4	18	38
Mean	4.0±1.0	2.8±0.8	20.0±3.8	38.4±5.7

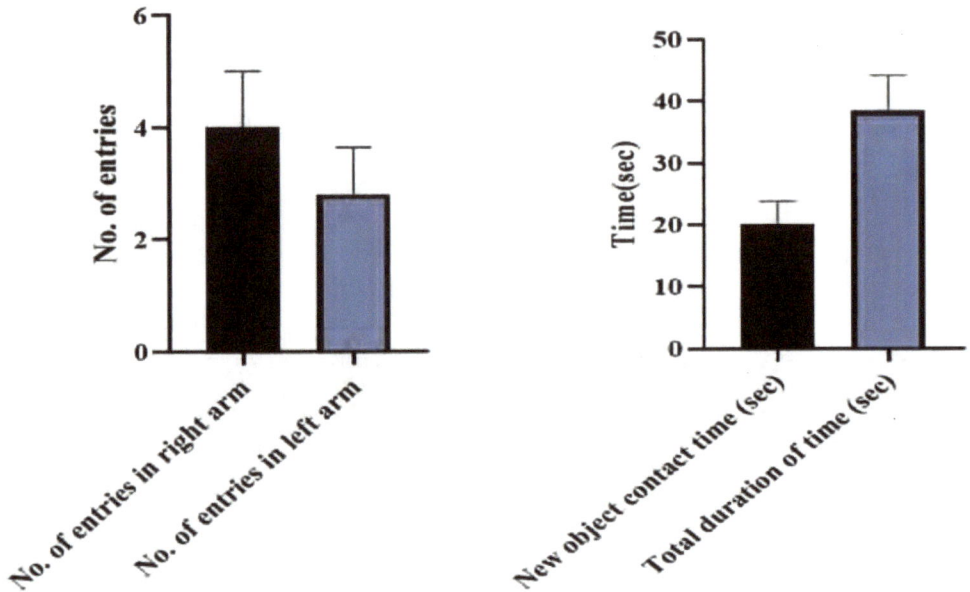

Statistical Analysis: Statistical analysis indicates that the number of entries into the right arm increases while the number of entries into the left arm decreases. Additionally, the contact time with the new object is approximately half of the total duration.

Applications for T-maze Test

The T-maze test is a widely used experimental paradigm in behavioral neuroscience and psychology. Its applications for T-maze are the following:

1. To assess spatial learning and memory
2. Decision making
3. Learning and cognitive flexibility
4. Neuropharmacology and neurological disorders
5. Anxiety and stress responses
6. Developmental studies

Y-MAZE TEST

A Y-shaped maze is used to measure Zebrafish preference for novel areas or spaces to evaluate spatial recognition and recall. The Y-maze is described in Fig. **(18.2)**.

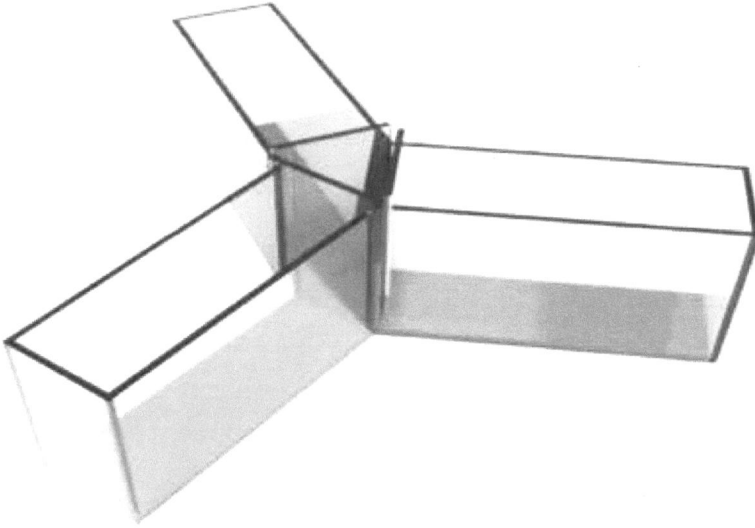

Fig. (18.2). Y-maze test apparatus.

Requirements

Animal: Adult Zebrafish

Equipment: Y-maze apparatus, Any maze software, Graph pad prism, Camera.

Procedure

1. The Y-Maze is a three-armed, symmetrical, capital "Y"-shaped tank. The normal dimensions of the arms are 25 cm long, 8 cm wide, and 15 cm high. The fish are free to swim around in the water that fills the tank.
2. Zebrafish are placed in the Y-Maze and given an appropriate amount of time to explore the tank. In response to both novelty and training-test intervals for spatial memory, the fish often spend more time in the novel arm than in the other arms.

A camera records the fish's behavior and measures the amount of time it spends in each arm, the total distance it travels, its mean speed, its turn angle, and the number of times it crosses a line. The fish's degree of spatial memory and exploratory behavior is evaluated using these measurements.

Observation

A dummy analysis is given in Table **18.2**.

Table 18.2. Observation table of the time spent on each arm and the no. of times lines are crossed on the T-maze apparatus of Zebrafish.

S. No.	Time Spent in Each Arm (Sec)			No. of Times Lines are Crossed
	Arm A	Arm B	Arm C	
1.	6	5	8	2
2.	8	8	9	2
3.	7	6	8	2
4.	9	7	7	2
5.	6	7	5	2
Mean	7.2±1.3	6.6±1.1	7.4±1.5	2.0±0.0

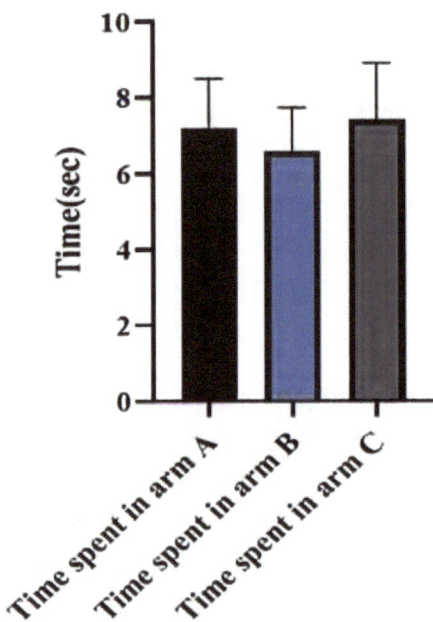

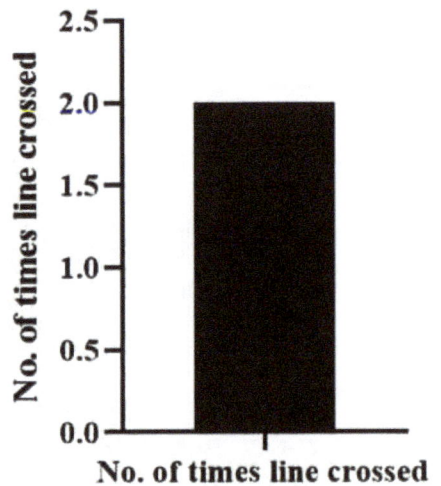

Statistical Analysis: Statistical analysis indicates that the time spent in arm B is less than arm A and arm C.

How is it different from T-maze?

Although both the Y maze and the T maze are commonly used in behavioral neuroscience, the designs they use and the cognitive processes they evaluate are different. The key differences are:

1. **Task Type:** T-maze involves a learned discrimination task (choosing between two spatial arms based on reward), while Y-maze involves spontaneous alternation behavior (choosing between three arms based on exploration).
2. **Cognitive Functions:** T-maze tests assess spatial learning, memory, and behavioral flexibility. Y-maze primarily tests short-term spatial working memory and exploratory behavior.

Experimental Setup: T-maze often requires training and specific reward-based protocols. Y-maze allows for spontaneous exploration without specific training.

Pros and cons of Y-maze over T-maze

The following are a few pros and cons of Y-mazes over T-mazes:

Pros

1. **Simplicity of task:** The task design of the Y-maze is less complicated than that of the T-maze. Usually, it involves alternating behavior that occurs on its own without the need for intensive conditioning or training. Free exploration of the maze by the animals can lessen the impact of stress related to training regimens.
2. **Assessment of spontaneous behavior:** The Y-maze evaluates spontaneous alternation, a trait that is indicative of exploratory and short-term working memory in space. This can reveal details about the animal's innate ability to investigate novel surroundings and make impulsive choices.
3. **Suitable for quick assessments:** Y-maze testing can be relatively quick, allowing researchers to assess multiple animals in a short amount of time. This can be advantageous for screening experiments or when evaluating large cohorts of animals.
4. **Minimal training required:** The Y-maze usually does not require substantial training, in contrast to the T-maze, which frequently requires training for animals to learn a specific task (*e.g.*, spatial discrimination). This may reduce experimental protocols and lessen the variance in outcomes based on learning curves.

Cons

1. **Limited cognitive assessment:** The Y-maze is mostly used to evaluate exploratory activity and spontaneous alternation behavior. Compared with the T-maze, which measures spatial discrimination and behavioral flexibility, it might not offer accurate insights into certain areas of learning, memory, or decision-making.

2. **Less control over experimental variables:** Since the Y-maze relies on spontaneous behavior, there is less control over the exact conditions under which animals make decisions. This can introduce variability in results and make it challenging to isolate specific cognitive processes or behaviors.
3. **Less versatile:** The Y-maze may not be suitable for certain types of experiments that require specific training protocols or more complex behavioral assessments. For example, studies focusing on reward-based learning or behavioral flexibility may benefit more from the T-maze design [4].

NOVEL TANK TEST

The tank is divided into two segments and used to measure the time spent in each part to measure locomotor activity and anxiety-like behavior. The novel tank test is described in Fig. (**18.3**).

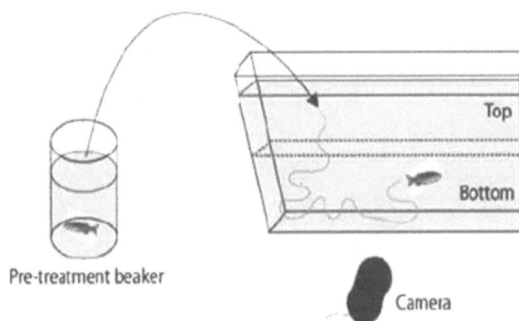

Fig. (18.3). Novel tank test apparatus.

Requirements

Animal: Adult Zebrafish

Equipment: Novel tank apparatus, Any maze software, Graph pad prism, Camera.

Procedure

1. To reduce stress, Zebrafish are allowed to get used to the lab environment for a certain amount of time before the test.
2. After being gently netted, the fish is moved to the novel tank, which is usually a clear tank with sections labeled top, middle, and bottom.
3. For five to ten minutes, use a camera to record the behavior of the fish.
4. Utilizing software, the captured video is examined to measure variables such as freezing behavior, locomotor activity, and the amount of time spent in each zone.

Zebrafish dive to the bottom when they are first brought to the new tank, and with time, they begin to explore the vertical space more. This steady increase in curiosity is thought to represent a decrease in anxiety.

Observation

A dummy analysis is given in Table **18.3**.

Table 18.3. Observation table of time spent and no. of entries in the top and bottom zone of the Novel tank test apparatus of Zebrafish.

S. No.	Time Spent in the Top Zone (Sec)	Time Spent in the Bottom Zone (Sec)	No. of Entries in the Top Zone	No. of Entries in the Bottom Zone
1.	15	38	3	10
2.	10	49	3	11
3.	16	35	5	9
4.	18	41	4	10
Mean	14.75±3.4	40.75±6.0	3.75±0.9	10±0.8

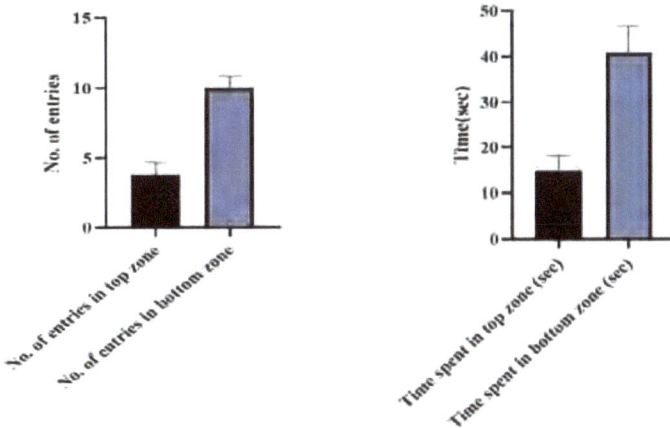

Statistical Analysis: Statistical analysis indicates that the number of entries and time spent in the top zone decrease, while the number of entries and time spent in the bottom zone increase.

Applications for Novel Tank Test

The novel tank test can be used in the following ways:

1. Assessment of anxiety-like behavior
2. Screening for anxiolytic and anxiogenic compounds
3. Stress response studies

4. Genetic and environmental manipulations
5. Developmental studies
6. Behavioral phenotyping [5]

INHIBITORY AVOIDANCE TEST

A learning and memory retention test that counts the amount of time spent in a particular location after a negative experience. The inhibitory avoidance test is described in Fig. (**18.4**).

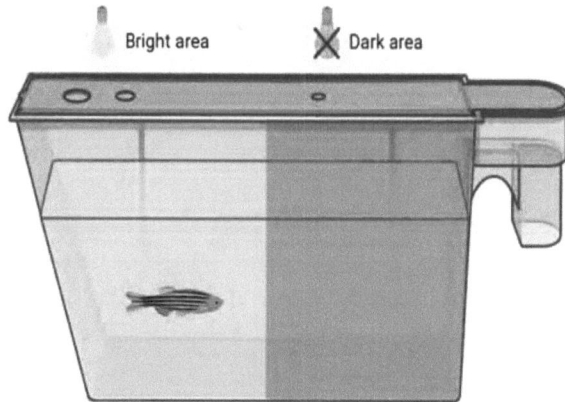

Fig. (18.4). Inhibitory avoidance test apparatus.

Requirements

Animal: Adult Zebrafish

Equipment: Avoidance test apparatus, Any maze software, Graph pad prism, Camera.

Procedure

1. To reduce environmental stress, introduce the Zebrafish to the test tank without any objects for three consecutive days.
2. Zebrafish are placed in a black and white box with a sliding door. The fish can swim from the white to the black compartment when the door is lifted. After entering the dark chamber, the fish is shocked with electricity (between 1-3 volts). To make sure the fish learns to associate the dark container with the shock, this procedure is performed once.
3. When the fish returns to the black-white box on the next day, the latency to enter the black compartment is assessed. Elevated latencies indicate enhanced learning of avoidance.
4. A camera records the test, and a measurement is made of the time it takes to

enter the black container. This test is designed to evaluate the fish's degree of inhibitory avoidance learning.

Observation

A dummy analysis is given in Table **18.4**.

Table 18.4. Observation table of time spent and no. of entries in bright and dark areas of the avoidance test apparatus of Zebrafish.

S. No.	No. of Entries in the Bright Area	No. of Entries in the Dark Area	Time Spent in Bright Areas (Sec)	Time Spent in Dark Areas (Sec)
1.	15	14	31	35
2.	12	10	28	30
3.	17	9	34	24
4.	19	7	39	21
Mean	15.75±2.9	10.0±2.9	33.0±4.6	27.50±6.2

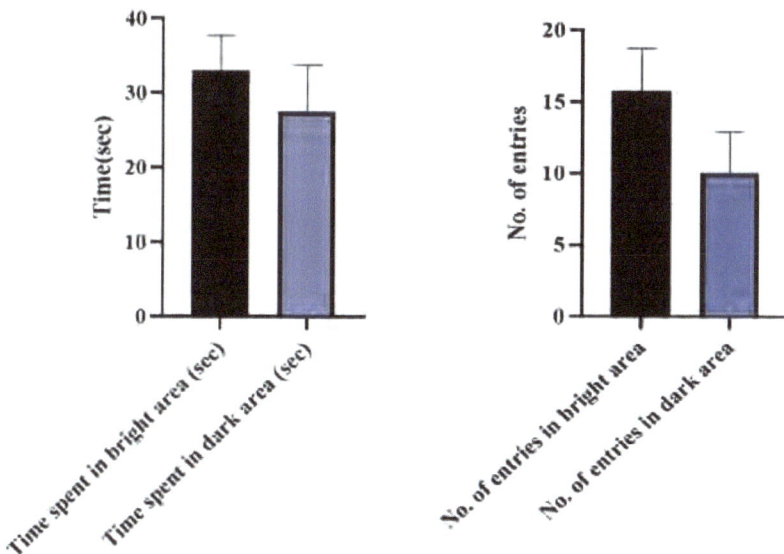

Statistical Analysis: Statistical analysis indicates that time spent and the number of entries are more in bright areas as compared to dark areas.

Applications of Inhibitory Avoidance Test

Here are several applications of the inhibitory avoidance test in research:

1. Fear memory and learning
2. Contextual fear conditioning

3. Assessment of memory consolidation
4. Pharmacological studies (*e.g.*, anxiety disorders)
5. Genetic and neurobiological research
6. Behavioral phenotyping [6]

LOCOMOTOR ACTIVITY TEST

A test that measures the speed and distance covered by Zebrafish to evaluate locomotor activity. The Locomotor Activity test is described in Fig. (**18.5**).

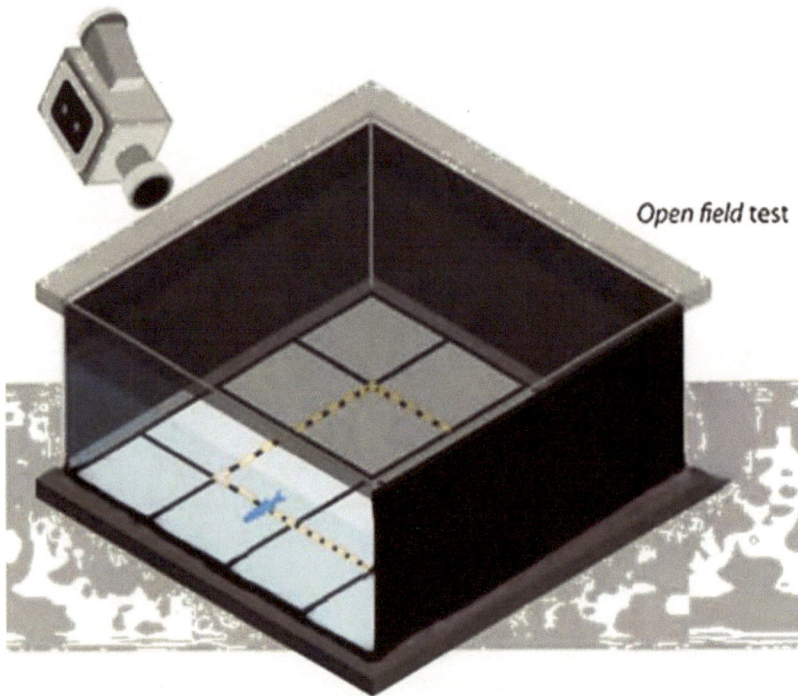

Open field test

Fig. (18.5). Open field Test Apparatus.

Requirements

Animal: Adult Zebrafish

Equipment: Open field test apparatus, Any maze software, Graph pad prism, Camera.

Procedure

1. To reduce stress, Zebrafish are allowed to be introduced to the experimental chamber for a predetermined amount of time before the test.

2. Zebrafish are arranged with a video-tracking system in a comparable container. The fish are free to swim around in the water.
3. The locomotor activity of the Zebrafish is captured with a camera or a video-tracking device. Usually, the recording lasts between 5 and 30 minutes.
4. Software is used to analyze the captured video to quantify variables such as velocity, distance traveled, and movement duration. These measurements are used to evaluate the locomotor activity.
5. A camera records the test, and a measurement is made of the time it takes to enter the black container. This test is designed to evaluate the fish's degree of inhibitory avoidance learning.

Observation

A dummy analysis is given in Table **18.5**.

Table 18.5. Observation table of parameters of the open field test apparatus of Zebrafish.

S. No.	No. of Times Lines are Crossed in 5 Mins	Time Spent on Corners (Sec)	Freezing Behavior (Sec)	Mirror Biting
1.	10	100	50	5
2.	8	120	40	6
3.	12	110	50	4
4.	11	100	30	5
Mean	10.25±1.7	107.5±9.5	42.50±9.5	5.0±0.8

Applications for Locomotor Activity Test

1. Neurological disorders such as Parkinson's disease or Huntington's disease
2. Behavioral studies
3. Circadian rhythm and sleep studies
4. Anxiety and depression [7]

APPLICATIONS

The learning test in Zebrafish has several applications:

1. **Studying neurodegenerative diseases:** Neurodegenerative disorders, including Parkinson's and Alzheimer's, are modeled in Zebrafish, and their effects on cognitive function are evaluated through learning tests.
2. **Pharmacological screening:** Learning tests are used to identify neurotoxic and neuroprotective substances that affect Zebrafish memory and learning.
3. **Genetic manipulation:** Learning tests are used to investigate the genetic basis

of memory and learning in Zebrafish, which are genetically manipulable.

4. **Behavioral neuroscience:** Behavioural neuroscience, including anxiety-like behaviors and locomotor activity in Zebrafish, is studied using learning tests.

5. **Cognitive research:** Cognitive functions like associative learning, object recognition, and spatial recognition are studied in Zebrafish.

6. **High-throughput screening:** In high-throughput screening, learning tests are employed to find novel chemicals that impact Zebrafish memory and learning.

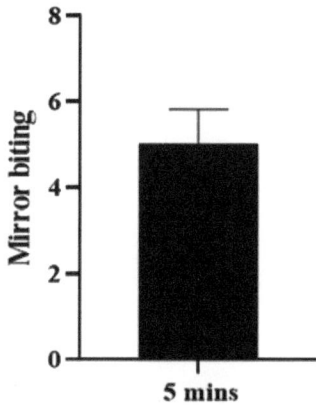

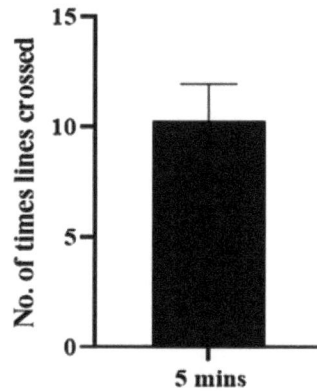

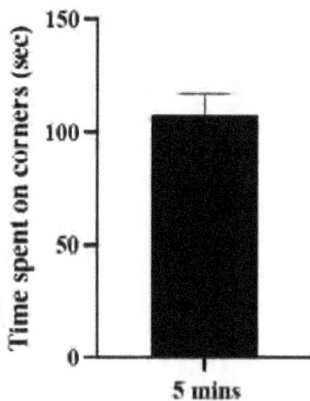

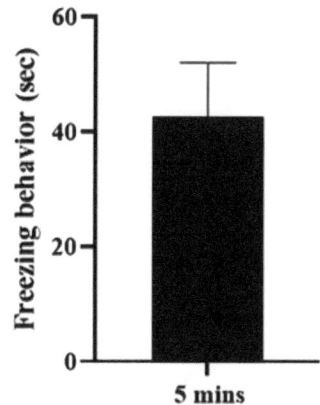

ADVANTAGES OF LEARNING TESTS

For research on learning and memory, the Zebrafish learning test has the following advantages:

1. **Genetic manipulation:** Zebrafish are excellent for researching the genetic basis of learning and memory because they are susceptible to genetic manipulation.

2. **Pharmacological screening:** Pharmacological screening using Zebrafish is done to find neurotoxic and neuroprotective substances that impact memory

and learning.

3. **Low maintenance costs:** Compared to other animal models, Zebrafish require less maintenance.
4. **Automated testing:** Automation can boost efficiency and throughput for some learning tests, such as the latent learning paradigm.
5. **Adaptability:** Zebrafish research has effectively adopted several learning paradigms from rodent studies, including those that use mazes.
6. **Behavioral tracking:** Measuring Zebrafish behaviors factors like swimming velocity and path shape with video tracking software like EthoVision XT can reveal important details about their capacity for learning and memory.
7. **Transparency:** Zebrafish embryos are transparent, making it possible to directly observe tissue morphogenesis at the cellular level. This information is valuable for researching the neural mechanisms underlying learning and memory.

LIMITATIONS OF LEARNING TESTS

The Zebrafish learning test has several disadvantages.

1. **Limited complexity:** It is possibly limited for Zebrafish to simulate more complex learning and memory processes because their learning assessments are often simpler than those performed on rats.
2. **Limited types of memory:** Some types of memory, like working memory and episodic-like memory, are more difficult to test in animals and cannot be developed in Zebrafish.
3. **Limited genetic manipulation:** Although Zebrafish are genetically manipulable, it can be challenging to accurately alter genes or pathways due to the complexity of their genetic structure.
4. **Limited automation:** Although many learning assessments can be automated, others would necessitate prolonged and labor-intensive training, which could restrict their application in high-throughput screening.
5. **Limited translational value:** Zebrafish learning tests may not be directly applicable to human learning and memory processes, which may restrict their application in diagnosing and treating cognitive issues in humans [8].

PRACTICE QUESTIONS

1. What do you understand by learning tests?
2. Discuss the effect of animal sex on learning tests.
3. What are the purposes of learning tests?
4. How each learning test is different from another?

REFERENCES

[1] Tan JK, Nazar FH, Makpol S, Teoh SL. Zebrafish: A pharmacological model for learning and memory research. Molecules 2022; 27(21): 7374.
[http://dx.doi.org/10.3390/molecules27217374] [PMID: 36364200]

[2] Gerlai R. Learning and memory in zebrafish (*Danio rerio*). Methods Cell Biol 2016; 134: 551-86.
[http://dx.doi.org/10.1016/bs.mcb.2016.02.005] [PMID: 27312505]

[3] Ngoc Hieu BT, Ngoc Anh NT, Audira G, *et al.* Development of a modified three-day T-maze protocol for evaluating learning and memory capacity of adult zebrafish. Int J Mol Sci 2020; 21(4): 1464.
[http://dx.doi.org/10.3390/ijms21041464] [PMID: 32098080]

[4] Galstyan DS, Kolesnikova TO, Kositsyn YM, *et al.* Cognitive tests in zebrafish (*Danio rerio*): T- and Y-mazes. Reviews on Clinical Pharmacology and Drug Therapy 2022; 20(2): 163-8.
[http://dx.doi.org/10.17816/RCF202163-168]

[5] Muralidharan A, Swaminathan A, Poulose A. Deep learning dives: Predicting anxiety in zebrafish through novel tank assay analysis. Physiol Behav 2024; 287: 114696.
[http://dx.doi.org/10.1016/j.physbeh.2024.114696] [PMID: 39293590]

[6] Manuel R, Gorissen M, van den Bos R. Relevance of test-and subject-related factors on inhibitory avoidance (performance) of zebrafish for psychopharmacology studies. Curr Psychopharmacol 2016; 5(2): 152-68.
[http://dx.doi.org/10.2174/2211556005666160526111427]

[7] Padilla S, Hunter DL, Padnos B, Frady S, MacPhail RC. Assessing locomotor activity in larval zebrafish: Influence of extrinsic and intrinsic variables. Neurotoxicol Teratol 2011; 33(6): 624-30.
[http://dx.doi.org/10.1016/j.ntt.2011.08.005] [PMID: 21871562]

[8] Vaz R, Hofmeister W, Lindstrand A. Zebrafish models of neurodevelopmental disorders: Limitations and benefits of current tools and techniques. Int J Mol Sci 2019; 20(6): 1296.
[http://dx.doi.org/10.3390/ijms20061296] [PMID: 30875831]

CHAPTER 19

Native Area Recognition Test in Zebrafish

Pratyush Porel[1], **Falguni Goel**[1] and **Shamsher Singh**[1,*]

[1] *Neuropharmacology Division, Department of Pharmacology, ISF College of Pharmacy, Moga, Punjab 142001, India*

INTRODUCTION

Aim: The aim of this chapter is to check the social interaction or social activity of an adult Zebrafish.

Scope and outcomes: The native area recognition test is a neurobehavioral test that may help evaluate those factors that may affect the social behavior and memory of Zebrafish in the lab as well as look at the potential translational effects of hormones, medicines, and other medical interventions. In the pursuit of a reliable Zebrafish model for psychiatric as well as neurodevelopmental disorders in humans with social deficits, this social preference test can prove to be beneficial.

Theory: The term "memory" is defined as the ability to recall or recognize a past after receiving stimuli in any one of the forms of visual, taste, smell, sound, touch, *etc* [1]. The native area recognition test is nothing but a test of cognition where the stimuli are present in the form of vision. Diagrammatically, the concept of study and native areas is illustrated in Fig. (**19.1**). To check the ability of the subject to distinguish the presence or absence of visual stimuli and the movement followed by them is the prime goal of the study. During the experiment, any other external clues should be avoided to provide a uniform and neutral experimental condition [2].

NATIVE AREA RECOGNITION TEST APPARATUS

The apparatus is made up of rectangular-shaped plexiglass with a length of 30 cm, a width of 22 cm, and a height of 11 cm. The reasons behind selecting plexiglass as a constructive material are its inertness to chemicals, non-toxic nature, good quality, and high level of transparency. The original chamber is divided into two equal chambers by

* **Corresponding author Shamsher Singh:** Neuropharmacology Division, Department of Pharmacology, ISF College of Pharmacy, Moga, Punjab 142001, India; Tel: +91-9779980588; E-mail: shamshersinghbajwa@gmail.com

a divider with a diameter of 4 cm, which is also made of plexiglass. The left-hand chamber, or floral chamber, was recently made, like the larger tank, where the fish belongs, and another part is left vacant and termed an empty chamber. There is sufficient water level for the fish to swim, and they can migrate to any of the two zones according to their interests. A camera is placed to record the video during the experiment with a holding stand, which is tightly attached to the tank wall through a clamp. The upper side tank is open, and it is used to introduce the experimental animal inside the apparatus. Now, the entire setup, as diagrammatically represented in Fig. (**19.2**), is ready to experiment [3].

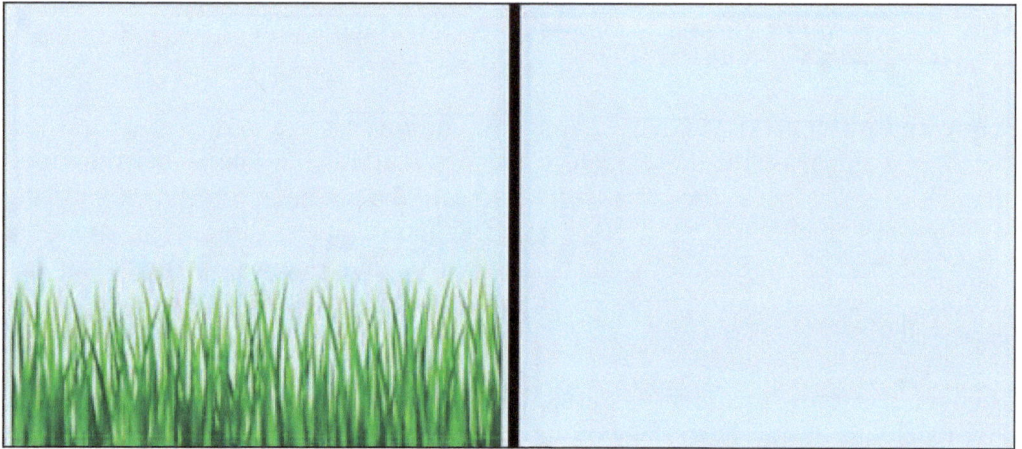

Fig. (19.1). Diagram illustrating the native area recognition.

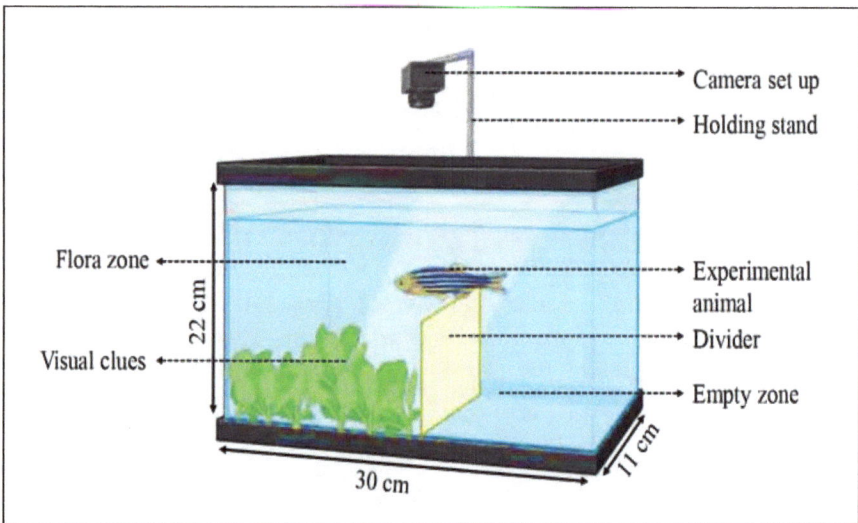

Fig. (19.2). Experimental setup for native area recognition test.

Features of the Apparatus

1. Shape: Rectangular
2. Length: 30 cm
3. Width: 11 cm
4. Height: 22 cm
5. Material: Plexiglass

ANY-maze Software

To make the study more scientific and reproducible, nowadays, researchers are highly aware of man-made mistakes. In the era of computer science and developmental technology, along with artificial intelligence, numerous applications are available on networking sites to make research more precise.

ANY-maze is a type of computational application with multidirectional features like video tracking, data analysis, solving mathematical equations, data transfer, and so many more. This application can be used to perform almost all behavioral tests, including Morris water maze, open field, Y-maze, T-maze, plus-maze, radial arm maze, forced swim test, *etc*. Due to its lower price, ease of operation, and, most importantly, multipurpose use, it is undoubtedly a promising software to be used in experimental pharmacology and enhances its acceptance among researchers throughout the world.

REQUIREMENTS

Animal: Adult Zebrafish

Equipment: Native area recognition apparatus, Any-maze software, Graph-pad-prism, Camera

PROCEDURE

Preparation of the Setup

1. Select one healthy fish from the larger tank and transfer it carefully into a smaller tank with the help of a net.
2. Keep the fish inside the small tank for 10 minutes to habituate itself to the environment.
3. Keep silence in the experimental room and avoid any other external stimuli such as an extra source of light, vibration, *etc*.
4. Maintain the temperature and humidity of the room throughout the experiment and provide a uniform experimental condition.
5. Properly clean the glass tank and apparatus with plenty of water and keep it

under a UV source for drying.

6. Fix a camera with a metal stand attached to the apparatus to record the movement of the fish inside the test apparatus at the best focal distance. This setup allows changing the position of the camera from the water level when required.

7. Turn on the software on the desktop before the start of the experiment and ensure that the application is running properly. There should be a strong network connection during the experiment.

Testing Procedure

1. After a habituation period of 10 minutes, the fish is introduced into the native area recognition apparatus, which is partially divided into two parts: one part of the apparatus is like the larger tank, and the other one lacks visual clues.

2. Allow the fish to settle inside the apparatus before testing for 1-2 minutes. With proper handling, try to keep the fish in a stress-free condition.

3. Turn on the camera and allow it to record the movement of the fish for the next 10 minutes.

4. Run on the ANY-maze software to track the movement of the fish. Notice the exploration behavior of the fish from a distance.

5. Stop the recording after the completion of the experiment and save the video for data analysis.

6. Take the fish out of the apparatus and place it in the smaller tank again for 30 minutes to rest between two or more consecutive tests.

Data Analysis

1. Review the previously recorded video and determine the type of behavioral nature shown by the fish during the experiment.

2. Videos are recorded of all studies and analyzed in a spreadsheet.

3. Perform statistical evaluation to compare the obtained data about spending time in the flora zone (known zone) and the empty zone (unknown zone).

4. Data should be checked by two independent study coordinators to keep the study from bias and produce more scientific as well as relevant data from the experiment.

Evaluation Criteria Duration in Every Zone

1. The quantity of time Zebrafish spend in the known (native) environment as opposed to the unfamiliar area serves as the main indicator. Spending more time in one's home region indicates familiarity with and a fondness for it.

2. **Investigative conduct:** The quantity and pattern of exploratory behavior, including the frequency of crossings across zones and the number of entrances

into distinct zones, are investigated. A greater amount of investigation in the new field may be a sign of curiosity and mental adaptability.

3. **Time lag to access a new area:** It is the amount of time it takes Zebrafish to go from being exposed to the test environment to the new region. An extended delay may indicate a predilection for the familiar surroundings and even apprehension about the new environment.

4. **Returns to the native region:** Zebrafish many times visit their home range after venturing into a new one. Regular returns might suggest a strong liking and recognition of the familiar surroundings.

5. **Patterns of movement:** Using tracking software to analyze movement patterns in detail may provide information on exploration methods and spatial memory. This covers route length, velocity, and certain actions such as wall-hugging or thigmotaxis.

6. **Evolution of behavior over time:** Learning and memory retention may be better understood by tracking how behavior changes throughout many trials. Learning is shown by a gradual gain in comfort or habit in the new environment.

OBSERVATION

The observation parameters (a dummy analysis) are described in Table **19.1**.

Table 19.1. Observation table of social behavior and memory by evaluation in native area recognition apparatus.

No. of Study	Time spent in Flora zone (sec)	Time spent in Empty zone (sec)
01	420	180
02	387	213
03	351	249
04	336	264
05	311	289
Total time spent in each zone	1805	1195
Mean	361±42.96	239±42.64

Graphical Presentation of Observation Table

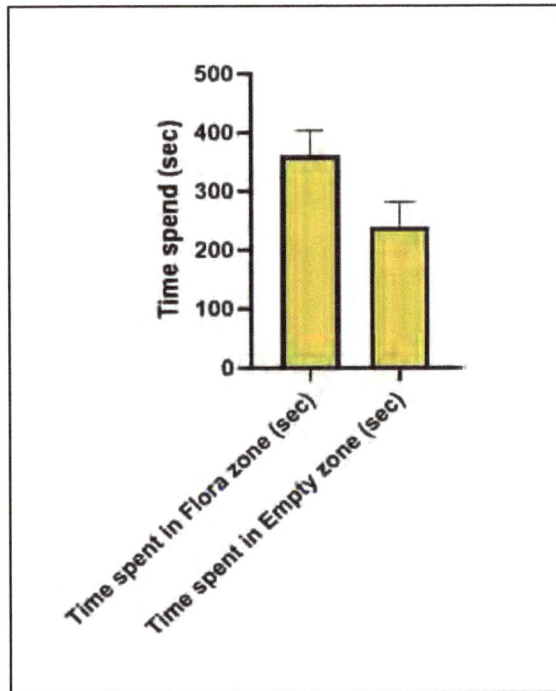

Statistical analysis: Statistical analysis shows that the time spent in the flora zone increased significantly than time spent in the empty zone.

RESULT

The Zebrafish rotation behavior test was understood and performed successfully, and the result indicates that there is a significant difference between the time spent in the flora zone and the empty zone. The result depicts that the flora zone was made like the larger tank and the fish also spent more time in that particular zone. This means that there was a significant memory formation regarding the native area recognition.

APPLICATIONS OF NATIVE AREA RECOGNITION TEST IN DISEASE OUTCOMES

1. In various neurological disorders, such as anxiety, depression, epilepsy, Alzheimer's disease (AD), Parkinson's disease (PD), Huntington's disease (HD), Multiple sclerosis (MS), Traumatic brain injury (TBI), and Autism spectrum disorder (ASD), the ability to recognize objects is greatly altered. So, in the study of neurodegenerative diseases, a native area recognition test is

performed to check for cognitive impairment [4].

2. This test also carries significant optical testing parameters, including the presence and absence of optical clues inside the test apparatus.

3. Native area recognition test is also an application of the optokinetic responses of the testing animal. The neural pathway of optokinetics passes from the retina to ocular motor neurons through the lateral geniculate body, followed by the optical lobe and cerebellar flocculus. Neural damage in any of these neuronal pathways may cause alterations in animal responses [5].

4. Alteration in the result of the experiment implies dysregulation of various neurophysiological pathways, which is further responsible for the pathogenesis of disease.

ADVANTAGES

1. **Ecologically relevant**: By using Zebrafish to study innate spatial memory and exploration behavior, the test offers ecologically sound insights into their cognitive processes. This test is in line with the way Zebrafish naturally navigate their environment since they are required to identify and retain distinct regions of their home.

2. **Non-invasive:** The fish are not physically harmed or put under a lot of stress by the native region identification test. This is advantageous for upholding the Zebrafish's welfare and ethical guidelines for study.

3. **Measurable and repeatable:** The test offers precise, measurable data including the amount of time spent in familiar *vs.* unfamiliar places, the quantity of entries, and the latency to enter unfamiliar zones. The replicable nature of these measures makes it possible to analyze cognitive processes objectively.

4. **High throughput:** The native area identification test is suited for high-throughput screening due to its ease of use and effectiveness. It is possible to test many fish at once, which is very helpful for extensive research projects or the screening of pharmaceuticals.

5. **Versatility:** Different areas of cognitive function, including learning, memory retention, and spatial navigation, may be studied with this exam. It may also be used to evaluate the results of pharmaceutical treatments, environmental adjustments, and genetic mutations.

6. **Cost-effective:** A partitioned tank and rudimentary tracking software are among the relatively basic and affordable tools needed for the test. This means that a variety of labs with varying financial limitations may use it.

7. **Behavioral consistency:** Zebrafish provide dependable and consistent answers in the native area identification test, which improves the accuracy of the information gathered. When behavior patterns are consistent, it might be simpler to identify minute variations brought about by manipulations during

experiments.

8. **Studies on growth and genetics:** Zebrafish are a great model organism for investigating the genetic foundation of cognitive processes due to their quick growth and genetic tractability. Researchers may use the native area recognition test to investigate how certain genes affect learning and spatial memory.

9. **Applications in pharmacology:** Because the test is responsive to pharmacological treatments, researchers may assess how different substances affect cognitive functioning. This is very helpful in identifying possible treatment drugs for cognitive impairments.

10. **Fast data collection:** The test makes it possible to gather and analyze behavioral data quickly, which makes it possible to get findings quickly and, if necessary, make fast changes to the design.

LIMITATIONS

1. **Environmental sensitivity:** Strict control of experimental settings is necessary since differences in tank layout, illumination, and water quality might affect the results.

2. **Individual variability:** Variability may be introduced by variations in Zebrafish behavior among individuals, necessitating higher sample numbers for statistical analysis to be robust.

3. **Difficulties with interpretation:** Observed behavior might sometimes be unclear and uninterpretable, necessitating cautious interpretation to differentiate between general exploratory behavior, anxiety, and memory.

4. **Effects of habituation:** Exposure to the test setting regularly may cause habituation, which lowers the test's efficacy after many attempts.

5. **Restricted range:** Evaluates spatial memory and exploration primarily; other components of cognitive function or sophisticated learning processes may not be adequately captured.

PRACTICE QUESTIONS

1. Why is a novel area recognition test performed?
2. Briefly describe the native area recognition tank.
3. What are the applications of the test?
4. Enlist evaluation criteria. Discuss any two.
5. Discuss some advantages and drawbacks of the test.

REFERENCES

[1]   Mujawar S, Patil J, Chaudhari B, Saldanha D. Memory. Ind Psychiatry J 2021; 30 (Suppl. 1): S311-4.
       [http://dx.doi.org/10.4103/0972-6748.328839] [PMID: 34908719]

[2]   Roy T, Bhat A. Learning and memory in juvenile zebrafish: What makes the difference–population or

rearing environment. Ethology 2016; 122(4): 308-18.
[http://dx.doi.org/10.1111/eth.12470]

[3]   Gerlai R, Fernandes Y, Pereira T. Zebrafish (*Danio rerio*) responds to the animated image of a predator: Towards the development of an automated aversive task. Behav Brain Res 2009; 201(2): 318-24.
[http://dx.doi.org/10.1016/j.bbr.2009.03.003] [PMID: 19428651]

[4]   Tan JK, Nazar FH, Makpol S, Teoh SL. Zebrafish: A pharmacological model for learning and memory research. Molecules 2022; 27(21): 7374.
[http://dx.doi.org/10.3390/molecules27217374] [PMID: 36364200]

[5]   Ahmed F, Nair DS, Thomas BB. A new optokinetic testing method to measure rat vision. Journal of visualized experiments: JoVE. 2022 Jul 7(185).
[http://dx.doi.org/10.3791/63357]

CHAPTER 20

Visual Impairment Testing in Zebrafish Using Rotation Test Apparatus

Kousik Maparu[1] and **Shamsher Singh**[1,*]

[1] *Neuropharmacology Division, Department of Pharmacology, ISF College of Pharmacy, Moga, Punjab 142001, India*

INTRODUCTION

Aim: The aim of this chapter is to investigate visual impairments of adult mutant Zebrafish using a rotation test apparatus.

Scope and outcomes: This experimental technique allows us to examine abnormalities and levels of visual sensitivity. Adult mutant Zebrafish are often identified using the Zebra Rotation Test, which features two containers: a transparent inner container and an outer drum wrapped in white paper with black segments. With this configuration, adult mutant screening is made easier by being able to measure the rod and cone visual thresholds. Modifications to the test include adjustments to light intensity and changes to the dimensions of the equipment.

Theory: The Zebrafish Rotation Test, also known as the Adult Escape Response Test, is a critical behavioral assay for identifying vision abnormalities in adult mutant Zebrafish [1]. This test quantitatively evaluates visual sensitivity by measuring the absolute thresholds of the Zebrafish's rod and cone photoreceptors [2]. During this experiment, Zebrafish are placed in a stationary glass container encircled by a revolving drum coated with white paper and a black stripe that represents a predatory threat. As the drum rotates, the fish automatically gravitate towards an opaque post in the middle of the container to protect themselves from the black stripe. Researchers can evaluate their visual performance and gain insights regarding their visual acuity through this activity. The test further allows for the measurement of rod and cone threshold after light exposure and enables the study of dark adaptation by varying the intensity of the white light source.

* **Corresponding author Shamsher Singh:** Neuropharmacology Division, Department of Pharmacology, ISF College of Pharmacy, Moga, Punjab 142001, India; Tel: +91-9779980588; E-mail: shamshersinghbajwa@gmail.com

Features of the Apparatus

- Rotation range: 0-20 rpm
- Centre post diameter: 3 cm
- Main Rotating Chamber: 10 cm diameter, transparent
- Rotating drum: 15 cm diameter

Instrument Specifications

- This instrumental setup includes a circular, transparent container approximately 10 cm in diameter, surrounded by a rotating acrylic drum wrapped in white paper.
- The drum features a 5 x 5 cm black stripe designed to mimic a threatening stimulus. A central opaque post, about 3 cm in diameter, keeps fish from swimming across the midline inside the container.
- Illumination is provided from above by a white light source with adjustable intensity tailored to the equipment's requirements. The drum is rotated at 10 rpm by a motor connected *via* a belt mechanism.
- Zebrafish behavior is tracked and captured with video tracking software like Noldus EthoVision XT. With this configuration, scientists may examine the behavioral responses of Zebrafish to visual stimuli, gaining knowledge about their sensitivity to light and how they react to it in controlled environments. The Zebrafish rotation test apparatus is shown in Fig. (**20.1**).

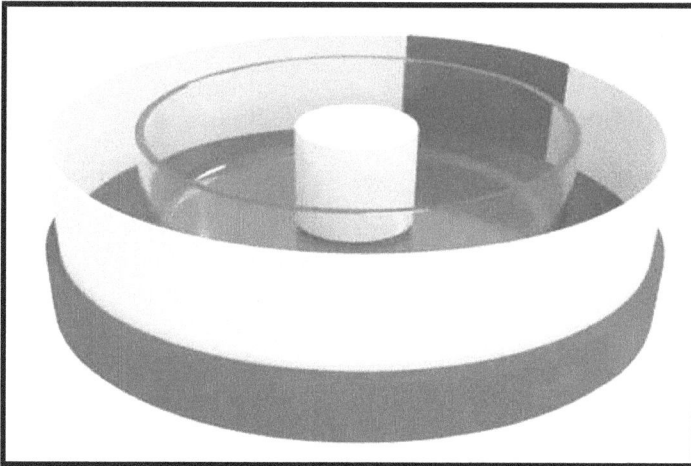

Fig. (20.1). Zebrafish rotation behaviour test apparatus.

REQUIREMENTS

Animal: Adult mutant Zebrafish

Instruments: Rotation test apparatus, Noldus EthoVision XT software.

PROCEDURE AND EVALUATION

Evaluation Method for Control Zebrafish

- **Housing:** Adult Zebrafish are individually housed in transparent containers before the experiment.
- **Light Adaptation:** Subjects undergo light adaptation by exposure to a bright light source emitting approximately 3.25×10^3 $\mu W/cm^2$ for about 20 minutes.
- **Dark Adaptation:** After light adaptation, the fish experience complete darkness (dark adaptation) for approximately 2 minutes.
- **Experiment Setup:** The fish are then introduced into the apparatus designed to assess their threshold light intensity for an escape response.
- **Light Intensity Adjustment:** Initially, the light intensity is set at log I = -3.0 and can be adjusted upwards in increments of 0.5 log units using neutral density filters on the drum [2].
- **Response Measurement:** If the fish do not respond to the initial intensity, the light intensity is increased by half a log unit until an escape response is observed.
- **Threshold Determination:** The lowest light intensity at which the fish exhibit an escape response is recorded as their absolute threshold.

Evaluation of Mutant Zebrafish

- **Mutant Screening Setup:** Light intensity is set to log I = -5.0 for screening mutants, which is approximately 1 log unit higher than the absolute rod threshold observed in wild-type Zebrafish. Individuals that do not exhibit the escape response at this intensity are segregated for further screening in subsequent days [2].
- **Generation of Mutant Individuals:** To generate mutant individuals, subjects undergo chemical mutagenesis using ENU (N-Ethyl-N-nitrosourea). Mutagenized individuals are then crossed with wild-type Zebrafish to produce the F1 generation.
- **Evaluation in F1 Generation:** In the F1 generation, individuals showing traits of night blindness are identified based on their behavior in the escape response test. These mutant individuals from the F1 generation are subsequently crossed with wild-type fish to produce the F2 generation.
- **Assessment in F2 Generation:** Both the F1 and F2 generations are examined to assess visual thresholds for both rods and cones using the escape response paradigm. This assessment helps in identifying and characterizing mutant Zebrafish with visual impairments across successive generations.

OBSERVATION

The observation parameters (a dummy analysis) are described in Table **20.1**.

Table 20.1. Observation table of visual impairments by evaluation in rotation test apparatus.

S. No.	Absolute Visual Threshold	
	Rods	Cones
Control	-4.5	-6
Mutant	-2.8	-3.9

Graphical Presentation of Observation Table

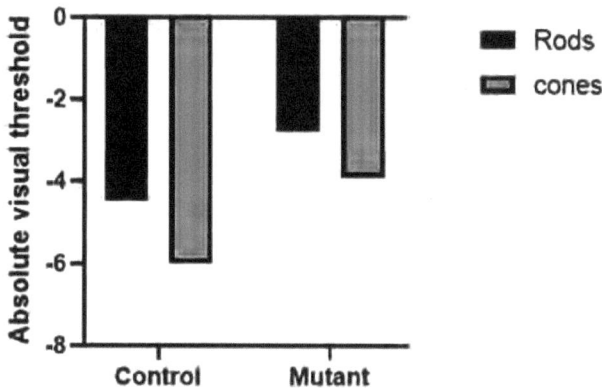

Statistical analysis: Statistical analysis shows that both the absolute threshold of cones and rods in mutant subjects are raised significantly.

RESULT

The Zebrafish rotation behavior test was understood and performed successfully, and the results of the observation table indicate that the sample data is depicted by comparing the absolute thresholds of the control and mutant subjects. It is evident from the graph that both the absolute threshold of cones and rods in mutant subjects are raised significantly.

APPLICATION

• The Zebrafish Rotation Behavior Test is a widely used method for categorizing adult mutant Zebrafish based on their visual abnormalities and sensitivity levels [3].

- Genetic screenings have employed this visual assessment to find mutations impairing the growth and operation of the visual system [4].

ADVANTAGES

- **Historical Significance:** The adult escape response model has a significant history and is the primary apparatus used to identify adult mutant Zebrafish based on visual defects.
- **Circadian Rhythms and Visual Sensitivity:** This method has shown a positive association between circadian rhythms and visual sensitivity.
- **Broad Applicability:** It is not limited to specific mutant strains like NBA; it has successfully identified numerous mutant strains with progressive retinal degeneration.
- **Relevance to Human Models:** These mutations are particularly relevant to human models as many outer retinal dystrophies in humans are progressive and predominantly affect elderly patients.

LIMITATIONS

The adult escape reaction task takes a long time to complete, and the experiment needs to be run by professionals.

PRACTICE QUESTIONS

- Describe the visual impairment test of Zebrafish.
- What is the Zebrafish rotation behavior test?
- What is the purpose of the Zebrafish rotation behavior test?
- What are the advantages of the Zebrafish rotation behavior test?
- Describe the evaluation methods of the Zebrafish rotation behavior test.

REFERENCES

[1]   Fleisch VC, Neuhauss SCF. Visual behavior in zebrafish. Zebrafish 2006; 3(2): 191-201.
[http://dx.doi.org/10.1089/zeb.2006.3.191] [PMID: 18248260]

[2]   Li L, Dowling JE. A dominant form of inherited retinal degeneration caused by a non-photoreceptor cell-specific mutation. Proc Natl Acad Sci USA 1997; 94(21): 11645-50.
[http://dx.doi.org/10.1073/pnas.94.21.11645] [PMID: 9326664]

[3]   Chhetri J, Jacobson G, Gueven N. Zebrafish—On the move towards ophthalmological research. Eye (Lond) 2014; 28(4): 367-80.
[http://dx.doi.org/10.1038/eye.2014.19] [PMID: 24503724]

[4]   Ganzen L, Venkatraman P, Pang C, Leung Y, Zhang M. Utilizing Zebrafish visual behaviors in drug screening for retinal degeneration. Int J Mol Sci 2017; 18(6): 1185.
[http://dx.doi.org/10.3390/ijms18061185] [PMID: 28574477]

Conclusion

In conclusion, this book has explored the multifaceted role of Zebrafish (*Danio rerio*) as a vital model organism in scientific research. From their unique biological characteristics and rapid developmental processes to their genetic similarities with humans, Zebrafish offer unparalleled opportunities for studying various aspects of biology and medicine. We examined key methodologies such as drug administration routes, blood collection techniques, and anaesthesia methods, emphasizing the importance of ethical considerations and welfare in experimental design. Behavioural assessments, including the Novel Diving Tank Test, Mirror Chamber Test, and various maze tests, have demonstrated Zebrafish's capacity to reveal insights into anxiety, memory, and social behaviour. These tests not only highlight the complexities of Zebrafish behaviour but also their utility in understanding neurological and psychological phenomena. This book serves as a foundation for exploring Zebrafish in diverse research contexts, encouraging the use of advanced imaging and genetic modifications to deepen our understanding of behaviour. By incorporating ecological factors and fostering interdisciplinary collaborations, researchers can further enhance the applications of Zebrafish in drug discovery and developmental biology.

By integrating these diverse topics, this book underscores the significance of Zebrafish in advancing our knowledge of developmental biology, pharmacology, and disease mechanisms. As research continues to evolve, Zebrafish will remain an invaluable asset in scientific inquiry, paving the way for breakthroughs in health and disease understanding. Their contributions to both basic and applied sciences ensure that they will be at the forefront of research for years to come.

Bibliography

Avdesh A, Chen M, Martin-Iverson MT, *et al.* Regular care and maintenance of a zebrafish (*Danio rerio*) laboratory: An introduction. J Vis Exp 2012; (69): e4196.
[PMID: 23183629]

Aleström P, D'Angelo L, Midtlyng PJ, *et al.* Zebrafish: Housing and husbandry recommendations. Lab Anim 2020; 54(3): 213-24.
[http://dx.doi.org/10.1177/0023677219869037] [PMID: 31510859]

Araujo-Silva H, Leite-Ferreira ME, Luchiari AC. Behavioral screening of alcohol effects and individual differences in Zebrafish (*Danio rerio*). Alcohol Alcohol 2020; 55(6): 591-7.
[http://dx.doi.org/10.1093/alcalc/agaa046] [PMID: 32533153]

Aoki R, Tsuboi T, Okamoto H. Y-maze avoidance: An automated and rapid associative learning paradigm in zebrafish. Neurosci Res 2015; 91: 69-72.
[http://dx.doi.org/10.1016/j.neures.2014.10.012] [PMID: 25449146]

Ahmad F, Richardson MK. Exploratory behaviour in the open field test adapted for larval zebrafish: Impact of environmental complexity. Behavioral processes 2013; Jan 1(92): 88-98.
[http://dx.doi.org/10.1016/j.beproc.2012.10.014]

Buske C. Zebrafish shoaling behavior: Its development, quantification, neuro-chemical correlates, and application in a disease model. Canada: University of Toronto 2013.

Burgess HA, Burton EA. A critical review of zebrafish neurological disease models− 1. The premise: Neuroanatomical, cellular and genetic homology and experimental tractability. Oxford Open Neuroscience. 2023;2:kvac018.

Balzarini V, Taborsky M, Wanner S, Koch F, Frommen JG. Mirror, mirror on the wall: The predictive value of mirror tests for measuring aggression in fish. Behav Ecol Sociobiol 2014; 68(5): 871-8.
[http://dx.doi.org/10.1007/s00265-014-1698-7]

Blaser RE, Peñalosa YM. Stimuli affecting zebrafish (*Danio rerio*) behavior in the light/dark preference test. Physiol Behav 2011; 104(5): 831-7.
[http://dx.doi.org/10.1016/j.physbeh.2011.07.029] [PMID: 21839758]

Basnet RM, Zizioli D, Taweedet S, Finazzi D, Memo M. Zebrafish larvae as a behavioral model in neuropharmacology. Biomedicines 2019; 7(1): 23.
[http://dx.doi.org/10.3390/biomedicines7010023] [PMID: 30917585]

Bailey JM, Oliveri AN, Levin ED. Pharmacological analyses of learning and memory in zebrafish (*Danio rerio*). Pharmacol Biochem Behav 2015; 139(0 0): 103-11.
[http://dx.doi.org/10.1016/j.pbb.2015.03.006] [PMID: 25792292]

Blaser RE, Vira DG. Experiments on learning in zebrafish (*Danio rerio*): A promising model of neurocognitive function. Neurosci Biobehav Rev 2014; 42: 224-31.
[http://dx.doi.org/10.1016/j.neubiorev.2014.03.003] [PMID: 24631853]

Braida D, Ponzoni L, Martucci R, Sparatore F, Gotti C, Sala M. Role of neuronal nicotinic acetylcholine receptors (nAChRs) on learning and memory in zebrafish. Psychopharmacology (Berl) 2013; 231.
[PMID: 24311357]

Choi TY, Choi TI, Lee YR, Choe SK, Kim CH. Zebrafish as an animal model for biomedical research. Exp Mol Med 2021; 53(3): 310-7.
[http://dx.doi.org/10.1038/s12276-021-00571-5]

Chaoul V, Dib EY, Bedran J, *et al.* Assessing drug administration techniques in zebrafish models of neurological disease. Int J Mol Sci 2023; 24(19): 14898.
[http://dx.doi.org/10.3390/ijms241914898] [PMID: 37834345]

Carradice D, Lieschke GJ. Zebrafish in hematology: Sushi or science? Blood 2008; 111(7): 3331-42.
[http://dx.doi.org/10.1182/blood-2007-10-052761] [PMID: 18182572]

Collymore C, Tolwani A, Lieggi C, Rasmussen S. Efficacy and safety of 5 anesthetics in adult zebrafish (*Danio rerio*). J Am Assoc Lab Anim Sci 2014; 53(2): 198-203.

Chen J, Tanguay RL, Simonich M, *et al.* TBBPA chronic exposure produces sex-specific neurobehavioral and social interaction changes in adult zebrafish. Neurotoxicol Teratol 2016; 56: 9-15.
[http://dx.doi.org/10.1016/j.ntt.2016.05.008] [PMID: 27221227]

Cognato GP, Bortolotto JW, Blazina AR, *et al.* Y-Maze memory task in zebrafish (*Danio rerio*): The role of glutamatergic and cholinergic systems on the acquisition and consolidation periods. Neurobiol Learn Mem 2012; 98(4): 321-8.
[http://dx.doi.org/10.1016/j.nlm.2012.09.008] [PMID: 23044456]

Dougnon G, Matsui H. Modelling autism spectrum disorder (ASD) and attention-deficit/hyperactivity disorder (ADHD) using mice and zebrafish. Int J Mol Sci 2022; 23(14): 7550.
[http://dx.doi.org/10.3390/ijms23147550] [PMID: 35886894]

Eissa MA, Abdullah R, Sharif F, Nasir MH. Repeated blood sampling from an adult *Danio rerio*. Zebrafish as a Model for Parkinson's disease.
[http://dx.doi.org/10.1201/9781003402893-7]

Fang L, Miller YI. Emerging applications for zebrafish as a model organism to study oxidative mechanisms and their roles in inflammation and vascular accumulation of oxidized lipids. Free Radic Biol Med 2012; 53(7): 1411-20.
[http://dx.doi.org/10.1016/j.freeradbiomed.2012.08.004] [PMID: 22906686]

Filik N, Vital A. Vital a fish: A critical review of zebrafish models in disease scenario and case reports screens. Laboratuvar Hayvanları Bilimi ve Uygulamaları Dergisi 2024; 4(2): 53-9.
[http://dx.doi.org/10.62425/jlasp.1426010]

Facciol A, Iqbal M, Eada A, Tran S, Gerlai R. The light-dark task in zebrafish confuses two distinct factors: Interaction between background shade and illumination level preference. Pharmacol Biochem Behav 2019; 179: 9-21.
[http://dx.doi.org/10.1016/j.pbb.2019.01.006] [PMID: 30699329]

Facciol A, Tran S, Gerlai R. Re-examining the factors affecting choice in the light–dark preference test in zebrafish. Behav Brain Res 2017; 327: 21-8.
[http://dx.doi.org/10.1016/j.bbr.2017.03.040] [PMID: 28359882]

Fontana BD, Cleal M, Parker MO. Female adult zebrafish (*Danio rerio*) show higher levels of anxiety-like behavior than males, but do not differ in learning and memory capacity. Eur J Neurosci 2020; 52(1): 2604-13.
[http://dx.doi.org/10.1111/ejn.14588] [PMID: 31597204]

Gerlai R. Zebrafish (*Danio rerio*): A newcomer with great promise in behavioral neuroscience. Neurosci Biobehav Rev 2023; 144: 104978.
[http://dx.doi.org/10.1016/j.neubiorev.2022.104978] [PMID: 36442644]

Gerlai RT. Relational learning in zebrafish: a model of declarative memory in humans? Behavioral and neural genetics of zebrafish. Academic Press 2020; pp. 205-20.
[http://dx.doi.org/10.1016/B978-0-12-817528-6.00013-9]

Gaspary KV, Reolon GK, Gusso D, Bonan CD. Novel object recognition and object location tasks in zebrafish: Influence of habituation and NMDA receptor antagonism. Neurobiol Learn Mem 2018; 155: 249-60.
[http://dx.doi.org/10.1016/j.nlm.2018.08.005] [PMID: 30086397]

Galstyan DS, Kolesnikova TO, Kositsyn YM, *et al.* Cognitive tests in zebrafish (*Danio rerio*): T- and Y-mazes. Reviews on Clinical Pharmacology and Drug Therapy 2022; 20(2): 163-8.
[http://dx.doi.org/10.17816/RCF202163-168]

Gerlai R, Fernandes Y, Pereira T. Zebrafish (*Danio rerio*) responds to the animated image of a predator: Towards the development of an automated aversive task. Behav Brain Res 2009; 201(2): 318-24.
[http://dx.doi.org/10.1016/j.bbr.2009.03.003] [PMID: 19428651]

Horzmann KA, Freeman JL. Making waves: New developments in toxicology with the zebrafish. Toxicol Sci 2018; 163(1): 5-12.
[http://dx.doi.org/10.1093/toxsci/kfy044] [PMID: 29471431]

Johnson A, Loh E, Verbitsky R, *et al.* Examining behavioural test sensitivity and locomotor proxies of anxiety-like behaviour in zebrafish. Sci Rep 2023; 13(1): 3768.
[http://dx.doi.org/10.1038/s41598-023-29668-9] [PMID: 36882472]

Kohale K. The housing and husbandry of zebrafish (*Danio rerio*) in a laboratory environment. Essentials of Laboratory Animal Science: Principles and Practices. 2021: 277-311.

Lucon-Xiccato T, Loosli F, Conti F, Foulkes NS, Bertolucci C. Comparison of anxiety-like and social behaviour in medaka and zebrafish. Sci Rep 2022; 12(1): 10926.
[http://dx.doi.org/10.1038/s41598-022-14978-1] [PMID: 35764691]

Li CY, Curtis C, Earley RL. Nonreversing mirrors elicit behaviour that more accurately predicts performance against live opponents. Anim Behav 2018; 137: 95-105.
[http://dx.doi.org/10.1016/j.anbehav.2018.01.010]

Levin ED, Cerutti DT. Behavioral Neuroscience of Zebrafish. In: Buccafusco JJ, Ed. Methods of Behavior Analysis in Neuroscience. 2nd ed., Boca Raton, FL: CRC Press/Taylor & Francis 2009.https://www.ncbi.nlm.nih.gov/books/NBK5216

Ma D, Zhang J, Lin H, Italiano J, Handin RI. The identification and characterization of zebrafish hematopoietic stem cells. Blood 2011; 118(2): 289-97.
[http://dx.doi.org/10.1182/blood-2010-12-327403] [PMID: 21586750]

Miller N, Greene K, Dydinski A, Gerlai R. Effects of nicotine and alcohol on zebrafish (*Danio rerio*) shoaling. Behav Brain Res 2013; 240: 192-6.
[http://dx.doi.org/10.1016/j.bbr.2012.11.033] [PMID: 23219966]

MacRae CA, Peterson RT. Zebrafish as a mainstream model for *in vivo* systems pharmacology and toxicology. Annu Rev Pharmacol Toxicol 2023; 63(1): 43-64.
[http://dx.doi.org/10.1146/annurev-pharmtox-051421-105617] [PMID: 36151053]

Muralidharan A, Swaminathan A, Poulose A. Deep learning dives: Predicting anxiety in zebrafish through novel tank assay analysis. Physiol Behav 2024; 287: 114696.
[http://dx.doi.org/10.1016/j.physbeh.2024.114696] [PMID: 39293590]

Magyary I. Floating novel object recognition in adult zebrafish: A pilot study. Cogn Process 2019; 20(3): 359-62.
[http://dx.doi.org/10.1007/s10339-019-00910-5] [PMID: 30810927]

May Z, Morrill A, Holcombe A, *et al.* Object recognition memory in zebrafish. Behav Brain Res 2016; 296: 199-210.
[http://dx.doi.org/10.1016/j.bbr.2015.09.016] [PMID: 26376244]

Maximino C, da Silva AWB, Gouveia A Jr, Herculano AM. Pharmacological analysis of zebrafish (*Danio rerio*) scototaxis. Prog Neuropsychopharmacol Biol Psychiatry 2011; 35(2): 624-31.
[http://dx.doi.org/10.1016/j.pnpbp.2011.01.006] [PMID: 21237231]

Manuel R, Gorissen M, van den Bos R. Relevance of test-and subject-related factors on inhibitory avoidance (performance) of zebrafish for psychopharmacology studies. Curr Psychopharmacol 2016; 5(2): 152-68.
[http://dx.doi.org/10.2174/2211556005666160526111427]

Maximino C, de Brito TM, da Silva Batista AW, Herculano AM, Morato S, Gouveia A Jr. Measuring anxiety in zebrafish: A critical review. Behav Brain Res 2010; 214(2): 157-71.
[http://dx.doi.org/10.1016/j.bbr.2010.05.031] [PMID: 20510300]

Miklósi Á, Andrew RJ. Right eye use associated with decision to bite in zebrafish. Behav Brain Res 1999; 105(2): 199-205.
[http://dx.doi.org/10.1016/S0166-4328(99)00071-6] [PMID: 10563493]

Nasiadka A, Clark MD. Zebrafish breeding in the laboratory environment. ILAR J 2012; 53(2): 161-8.
[http://dx.doi.org/10.1093/ilar.53.2.161] [PMID: 23382347]

Ngoc Hieu BT, Ngoc Anh NT, Audira G, *et al.* Development of a modified three-day T-maze protocol for evaluating learning and memory capacity of adult zebrafish. Int J Mol Sci 2020; 21(4): 1464.
[http://dx.doi.org/10.3390/ijms21041464] [PMID: 32098080]

Oliveira RF. Mind the fish: Zebrafish as a model in cognitive social neuroscience. Front Neural Circuits 2013; 7: 131.
[http://dx.doi.org/10.3389/fncir.2013.00131] [PMID: 23964204]

Ogi A, Licitra R, Naef V, *et al.* Social preference tests in zebrafish: A systematic review. Front Vet Sci 2021; 7: 590057.
[http://dx.doi.org/10.3389/fvets.2020.590057] [PMID: 33553276]

Ogi A, Licitra R, Naef V, *et al.* Social preference tests in zebrafish: A systematic review. Front Vet Sci 2021; 7: 590057.
[http://dx.doi.org/10.3389/fvets.2020.590057] [PMID: 33553276]

Pagnussat N, Piato AL, Schaefer IC, *et al.* One for all and all for one: The importance of shoaling on behavioral and stress responses in zebrafish. Zebrafish 2013; 10(3): 338-42.
[http://dx.doi.org/10.1089/zeb.2013.0867] [PMID: 23802189]

Polverino G, Abaid N, Kopman V, Macrì S, Porfiri M. Zebrafish response to robotic fish: Preference experiments on isolated individuals and small shoals. Bioinspir Biomim 2012; 7(3): 036019.
[http://dx.doi.org/10.1088/1748-3182/7/3/036019] [PMID: 22677608]

Reed B, Jennings M. Guidance on the housing and care of Zebrafish Southwater. Royal Society for the Prevention of Cruelty to Animals 2011.

Rihel J, Ghosh M. Zebrafish. Drug discovery and evaluation: pharmacological assays. Cham: Springer International Publishing 2016; pp. 4071-155.
[http://dx.doi.org/10.1007/978-3-319-05392-9_135]

Rowe CJ, Crowley-Perry M, McCarthy E, Davidson TL, Connaughton VP. The three-chamber choice behavioral task using zebrafish as a model system. J Vis Exp 2021; (170): e61934.
[PMID: 33938895]

Roy T, Bhat A. Learning and memory in juvenile zebrafish: what makes the difference–population or rearing environment. Ethology 2016; 122(4): 308-18.
[http://dx.doi.org/10.1111/eth.12470]

Stevens CH, Reed BT, Hawkins P. Enrichment for laboratory zebrafish—A review of the evidence and the challenges. Animals (Basel) 2021; 11(3): 698.
[http://dx.doi.org/10.3390/ani11030698] [PMID: 33807683]

Snekser JL, Ruhl N, Bauer K, McRobert SP. The influence of sex and phenotype on shoaling decisions in Zebrafish. Int J Comp Psychol 2010; 23(1)
[http://dx.doi.org/10.46867/IJCP.2010.23.01.04]

Sison M, Gerlai R. Associative learning in zebrafish (*Danio rerio*) in the plus maze. Behav Brain Res 2010; 207(1): 99-104.
[http://dx.doi.org/10.1016/j.bbr.2009.09.043] [PMID: 19800919]

Stefanello FV, Fontana BD, Ziani PR, Müller TE, Mezzomo NJ, Rosemberg DB. Exploring object discrimination in zebrafish: Behavioral performance and scopolamine-induced cognitive deficits at different retention intervals. Zebrafish 2019; 16(4): 370-8.
[http://dx.doi.org/10.1089/zeb.2018.1703] [PMID: 31145046]

Stewart AM, Gaikwad S, Kyzar E, Kalueff AV. Understanding spatio-temporal strategies of adult zebrafish exploration in the open field test. Brain Res 2012; 1451: 44-52.
[http://dx.doi.org/10.1016/j.brainres.2012.02.064] [PMID: 22459042]

Steenbergen PJ, Richardson MK, Champagne DL. Patterns of avoidance behaviours in the light/dark preference test in young juvenile zebrafish: A pharmacological study. Behav Brain Res 2011; 222(1): 15-25.
[http://dx.doi.org/10.1016/j.bbr.2011.03.025] [PMID: 21421013]

Teraoka H, Dong W, Hiraga T. Zebrafish as a novel experimental model for developmental toxicology. Congenit Anom (Kyoto) 2003; 43(2): 123-32.
[http://dx.doi.org/10.1111/j.1741-4520.2003.tb01036.x] [PMID: 12893971]

Tan JK, Nazar FH, Makpol S, Teoh SL. Zebrafish: A pharmacological model for learning and memory research. Molecules 2022; 27(21): 7374.
[http://dx.doi.org/10.3390/molecules27217374] [PMID: 36364200]

Von Krogh K, Higgins J, Saavedra Torres Y, Mocho JP. Screening of anaesthetics in adult zebrafish (*Danio rerio*) for the induction of euthanasia by overdose. Biology (Basel) 2021; 10(11): 1133.
[http://dx.doi.org/10.3390/biology10111133] [PMID: 34827125]

Varga ZK, Zsigmond Á, Pejtsik D, *et al.* The swimming plus-maze test: A novel high-throughput model for assessment of anxiety-related behaviour in larval and juvenile zebrafish (*Danio rerio*). Sci Rep 2018; 8(1): 16590.
[http://dx.doi.org/10.1038/s41598-018-34989-1] [PMID: 30410116]

Weber DN, Ghorai JK. Experimental design affects social behavior outcomes in adult zebrafish developmentally exposed to lead. Zebrafish 2013; 10(3): 294-302.
[http://dx.doi.org/10.1089/zeb.2012.0780] [PMID: 23672286]

Zang L, Shimada Y, Nishimura Y, Tanaka T, Nishimura N. Repeated blood collection for blood tests in adult zebrafish. J Vis Exp 2015; 102.

Zang L, Shimada Y, Nishimura Y, Tanaka T, Nishimura N. A novel, reliable method for repeated blood collection from aquarium fish. Zebrafish 2013; 10(3): 425-32.
[http://dx.doi.org/10.1089/zeb.2012.0862] [PMID: 23668933]

Zhang J, Liu M, Cui W, Yang L, Zhang C. Quercetin affects shoaling and anxiety behaviors in zebrafish: Involvement of neuroinflammation and neuron apoptosis. Fish Shellfish Immunol 2020; 105: 359-68.
[http://dx.doi.org/10.1016/j.fsi.2020.06.058] [PMID: 32693159]

SUBJECT INDEX

A

Abdominal cavity 18, 19
Abiotic factor 40, 41
Abnormalities 48, 53, 58, 135, 161, 164
  developmental 58
  disease-related cognitive 135
  dopamine function 53
  identifying vision 161
  metabolic 48
  visual 164
Absolute visual threshold 164
Acclimation period 107
Acrylic materials 101
Activity 9, 34, 71, 81, 86, 99, 105, 108, 122, 125, 136, 137, 142, 149, 152
  behaviors and locomotor 105, 149
  exploratory 99, 142
  free-swimming 9
  heightened 122
  metabolic 34
  neuronal 136, 137
  social 71, 86, 152
  spontaneous motor 125
  stress-induced 81
  vertical 108
Activity levels 96, 99
Acute 11, 42, 49
  administration 42
  kidney injury 49
  toxicity test 11
Adrenal insufficiency 49
Adult 17, 19, 20, 30, 37, 38, 62, 63, 76, 77, 87, 89, 101, 102, 107, 161, 162, 164, 165
  escape response model 165
  escape response test 161
  mutant Zebrafish 161, 162, 164, 165
  Zebrafish 17, 19, 20, 30, 37, 38, 62, 63, 76, 77, 87, 89, 101, 102, 107
  Zebrafish and larvae 38
Agrochemicals 9

Alcohol-disordered polarization 42
Alzheimer's disease 52, 118, 125, 130, 135, 157
Amyloid-beta proteins 135
Amyotrophic lateral sclerosis 49, 53
Anesthesia 32, 33, 34, 58
  inhalation 33, 34
  level of 32, 34
  providing 33
  repeated 58
    exploration 33
Animal models 7, 37, 38, 55
  alternative 7, 38
  novel 37
  preferred 55
Anti-HCV therapeutics 56
Antiepileptic drugs 17
Anxiety 64, 66, 72, 76, 80, 94, 92, 96, 98, 133
  anticipatory 76, 94
  assessing 64, 133
  diagnose 66
  heightened 80, 96
  monitor 98
  natural 92
  social 72
Artemia sp 4
Assays 9, 12, 21, 65, 87
Assessment 59, 66, 81, 86, 99, 131, 143, 165
  complex behavioral 143
  complicating dose-response 59
  quantitative 86
  rapid 66
  regular 81
  risk 99, 131
  visual 165
Atherosclerosis 49, 57
Atrial fibrillation 57
Autism spectrum disorders (ASD) 49, 53, 135, 157
Automated behavioral assay systems 136

B

Behavioural 38, 44, 65, 66, 86, 166
  assessments 86, 166
  changes 44
  ecology 65
  measure 38
  profile 66
  studies 38
  tests 65
Beta-amyloid plaques 52
Biomarkers 28, 51
Bradycardia 12

C

Canister filter 3
Capabilities 13, 101, 102, 103, 105
  decision-making 101, 102, 103, 105
  high-throughput 13
Cardiac puncture method 26
Cardiovascular 12, 49
  atrial fibrillation 49
  toxicity 12
Cerebellar flocculus 158
Chemotherapeutic agents 17
Ciliopathy 49
Circadian rhythm 148, 165
Clove Oil 32
Congenital 52
  cardiac defect 52
  cardiovascular abnormality 52
Context-dependent behavior 73
Contextual fear conditioning 146
Cushing's disease 49
Cypriniformes 1

D

DiGeorge Syndrome 52
Disorders 12, 28, 38, 48, 49, 52, 53, 60, 65,
    68, 69, 72, 83, 105, 118, 124, 125, 130,
    135, 139, 148, 152, 157
  anxiety-related 124
  autism spectrum 49, 53, 72, 135, 157
  haematological 28
  intestinal 12
  multifaceted behavioural 38
  neurodegenerative 52, 53, 105, 118, 130,
    148

  neurodevelopmental 69, 83, 152
  neurological 48, 60, 68, 125, 139, 148, 157
  stress-related 65
DNA 21, 28, 52
Dopaminergic 11, 53
  circuits 53
  neurons 11
Duchenne muscular dystrophy (DMD) 51

E

Electrocardiogram 57
Electrophysiological setups 136
Elevated 96, 145
  latencies 145
  thigmotaxis levels 96
Enhanced green fluorescent protein (EGFP)
    18
Epilepsy 39, 44, 125, 135, 157
Eppendorf tube 26
Equipment, video 89
Erythropoietic protoporphyria 52
Ethical 28, 35, 58, 74, 103, 112, 123, 158
  criteria 28
  guidelines 103, 123, 158
  implications 58
  practices 35
  questions 74
  standards 74, 112
Euthanasia 19, 32
Euthanize 19

F

Factors 28, 40, 42, 52, 65, 71, 78, 79, 81, 92,
    97, 107, 126, 166
  behavioral 92
  biotic 40, 42
  environmental 28, 71, 126
  external 81, 107
  genetic 65, 78, 97
  incorporating ecological 166
  transcription 52
Female Zebrafish 1, 5

G

GABAergic system 42
Genomic analyses 47

H

Haematocrit 28
Hepatic stellate cells (HSCs) 55
Hepatitis C virus (HCV) 56
Hepatocellular carcinoma 55
Herpes simplex virus (HSV) 56
Huntington's disease (HD) 49, 53, 118, 125, 130, 148, 157

I

Incubation chamber 6
Influenza A virus (IAV) 55
Injection procedure 19
Intrusive operations 23
Investigating obesity 50
Investigative 96, 155
  behaviour 96
  conduct 155

L

Labyrinth 94, 96
  cross-shaped 94
Larvae 6, 134
  sick 6
  transparent 134
  unhealthy 6
Light/dark cycles 137
Light-dark preference test 9
Liver sinusoidal endothelial cells (LSECs) 55
Lymphoid leukaemia 54

M

Maze test 96, 98, 101, 110, 166
  square 110
  apparatus 96
Melanocytes 54
Micro capillary tube 24
Miles-carpenter syndrome (MCS) 51
Multiple sclerosis (MS) 157
Mutant screening setup 163
Mutant Zebrafish 163
Mycobacterium marinum 55
Mycobacterium tuberculosis 55

N

Naturalistic behaviour 65
Nerve, optic 9
Neural crest progenitors (NCPs) 55
Neuropharmacology Division 1, 16, 23, 30, 37, 47, 62, 68, 76, 83, 87, 94, 101, 107, 115, 121, 127, 133, 152, 161
Neurotoxins 17
Neurotransmitter 44
Nitrification 3
Non-invasive methodologies 59
Noonan Syndrome 58
Novel object recognition test (NORT) 116
Novel tank diving 63

O

Open field apparatus (OFA) 115, 121, 122, 123, 124, 125
Operant 134
Operculum 20, 26
Optical lobe 158
Optokinetic assay 9
Osteoporosis 58
Oxidative stress 9

P

Parkinson's disease (PD) 49, 53, 118, 125, 130, 135, 148, 157
Photo-motor response assay 11
Phylogenetic divergence 47
Plexiglass doors 128
Plus-Maze test 94, 95, 97, 99
Protoporphyrin IX 52

Q

Quantitative analysis 86

R

Regenerative medicines 28
Resazurin 12
Restricted behavioral repertoire 92

S

Screening 142, 163
   experiments 142
   mutants 163
Square 107, 109, 111, 113
   cognitive maze (SCM) 107, 109
   -maze test 107, 109, 111, 113
Statistical analysis 64, 71, 72, 79, 85, 104,
      110, 118, 130, 139, 141, 144, 146, 157,
      164

T

Toxicity analysis 9
Transcriptional modifications 56
Transcriptomic analyses 54
Traumatic brain injury (TBI) 39, 44, 125, 133,
      157

U

Underwater conditions 62
UV filters 4
UV source 155

V

Variables 89, 92, 143
   environmental 92
   experimental 89, 143
Vascularization 9
Ventricular hypertrophy 58
Videos 103, 143, 148, 155
   captured 143, 148
   recorded 103, 155
Visual impairment test 165
Visual thresholds 161, 163

W

Wastewater 4

Y

Y-maze 101, 102, 104, 106, 136, 139, 140,
      142, 143, 154
   apparatus 104, 136, 140
   test in Zebrafish 101, 106

Z

Zebra 121, 136, 161
   box system 136
   lab 121
   rotation Test 161
Zone preferences 108

www.ingramcontent.com/pod-product-compliance
Lightning Source LLC
Chambersburg PA
CBHW041703210326
41598CB00007B/512